Life Course Research and Social Policies

Volume 4

Series editors
Laura Bernardi
Dario Spini
Michel Oris

Life course research has been developing quickly these last decades for good reasons. Life course approaches focus on essential questions about individuals' trajectories, longitudinal analyses, cross-fertilization across disciplines like life-span psychology, developmental social psychology, sociology of the life course, social demography, socio-economics, social history. Life course is also at the crossroads of several fields of specialization like family and social relationships, migration, education, professional training and employment, and health. This Series invites academic scholars to present theoretical, methodological, and empirical advances in the analysis of the life course, and to elaborate on possible implications for society and social policies applications.

More information about this series at http://www.springer.com/series/10158

Claudine Burton-Jeangros • Stéphane Cullati
Amanda Sacker • David Blane
Editors

A Life Course Perspective on Health Trajectories and Transitions

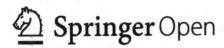

Editors
Claudine Burton-Jeangros
Swiss National Center of Competence
for Research LIVES – Overcoming
Vulnerability: Life Course Perspectives
University of Geneva
Geneva, Switzerland

Stéphane Cullati
Swiss National Center of Competence
for Research LIVES – Overcoming
Vulnerability: Life Course Perspectives
University of Geneva
Geneva, Switzerland

Amanda Sacker
ESRC International Centre for Life Course
Studies in Society and Health (ICLS)
University College London
London, UK

David Blane
ESRC International Centre for Life Course
Studies in Society and Health (ICLS)
University College London
London, UK

ISSN 2211-7776   ISSN 2211-7784 (electronic)
Life Course Research and Social Policies
ISBN 978-3-319-37244-0   ISBN 978-3-319-20484-0 (eBook)
DOI 10.1007/978-3-319-20484-0

Springer Cham Heidelberg New York Dordrecht London

Springer International Publishing AG Switzerland is part of Springer Science+Business Media (www.springer.com)

Contents

Chapter 1
Introduction

Claudine Burton-Jeangros, Stéphane Cullati, Amanda Sacker, and David Blane

The present volume contributes to life course research with a specific emphasis on health trajectories as they unfold along individual lives in specific socio-historical contexts. It brings together a range of contributions from different disciplines to shed light on the complex social and biological processes which influence people's health. The Introduction addresses the goals of life course epidemiology and the contribution which insights from the life course perspective can bring to the study of health. Theoretical, methodological and policy considerations associated with life course epidemiology are presented to discuss the current state of the field and expected developments to come. The Introduction finally presents the different contributions of this volume.

The Ambitions of Life Course Epidemiology

Health has been traditionally envisioned as a state, encompassing different dimensions along the lines of the World Health Organization's long-established definition: "[health is] a state of complete physical, mental and social wellbeing and not merely the absence of disease or infirmity" (WHO 1946). A recent discussion of the

C. Burton-Jeangros (✉) • S. Cullati
Swiss National Center of Competence for Research LIVES – Overcoming Vulnerability: Life Course Perspectives, University of Geneva, Geneva, Switzerland
e-mail: Claudine.jeangros@unige.ch; Stephane.cullati@unige.ch

A. Sacker • D. Blane
ESRC International Centre for Life Course Studies in Society and Health (ICLS), University College London, London, UK
e-mail: a.sacker@ucl.ac.uk; d.blane@imperial.ac.uk

© The Author(s) 2015
C. Burton-Jeangros et al. (eds.), *A Life Course Perspective on Health Trajectories and Transitions*, Life Course Research and Social Policies 4,
DOI 10.1007/978-3-319-20484-0_1

concept, raising the limitations of this definition, highlighted the dynamic nature of health by suggesting that it reflects "the ability to adapt and to self manage" (Huber et al. 2011, p. 1). This conception is fully in line with the life course perspective which is interested in understanding how the past influences the present. The dynamic component of health is further emphasized by the idea, promoted by epidemiological thinking, that it results from individual exposure to a range of risks. The combination of physiological and social resources that individuals can count on is expected to influence their ability to adapt, with responses ranging between vulnerability and resilience.

Examining health over time involves considering how individual trajectories unfold along different pathways. These trajectories can be stable, at different levels since some individuals remain in good health while others remain in poor health as years go by. Health trajectories can reflect a decline, as can be expected among the elderly who progressively lose functional and cognitive capacities, or alternatively indicate an improvement, for example among those who recover from a specific disease and its associated disability. Last but not least, these trajectories can fluctuate in an unclear trend among individuals who experience successive episodes of good and poor health. Health trajectories reflect continuous developments, informing on individual histories of health (Colerick Clipp et al. 1992). The notion of trajectories is therefore implying a long-term approach, in contrast with the idea of transition which is focused on short-term events or changes (Kuh et al. 2003). While trajectories are estimated from a succession of health measures, reported at more or less short intervals over time (a few days to several years), transitions measure changes between health states. Since these transitions can occur at the physiological level or in social circumstances, "life course epidemiology attempts to integrate biological and social risk processes" (Kuh et al. 2003, p. 778).

Interest in a life course perspective emerged in the 1980s in relation to chronic diseases (Aboderin et al. 2001; Kuh and Ben-Shlomo 2004; Wilkinson 1996). Converging research interests helped consolidate life course epidemiology over the last decade of the twentieth century, as an interdisciplinary field fostering collaborations between the natural and social sciences (Blane et al. 2007; Graham 2002). Expanding Elder's proposition that the individual life course is shaped by multiple trajectories (Elder 1998), it emphasizes the importance of understanding the interactions between biological change and social change at the individual level. This research studies human beings as both social and biological entities: social in the sense of their plasticity to material and cultural context; biological in the sense of development from a single newly-fertilised cell to the estimated 27.2 trillion cells of an adult who subsequently loses functional capacity, develops disease(s) and dies.

The integration of social and biological components in the study of health is a long-standing issue that has recently gained considerable attention (Anderson 1998; Blane et al. 2013; Glass and McAtee 2006). However life course epidemiology is truly innovative in that it addresses the complex interactions developing over time between a range of determinants and outcomes. Typical questions focus on the influence of social factors on health: How does social class get into the molecules, cells and tissues of the body to produce social class differences in life expectancy and cause of death? How does social participation enhance resilience at older ages? How does childhood experience of parental separation contribute to the later onset of anxiety and depression? However, reverse influences are also of interest: How does poor health during childhood restrict education opportunities and consequently professional paths? How does depression affect marital life? Considering that these contrasted influences interact, they are likely to produce distinct patterns of disadvantage or privilege. Therefore this research is not only interested in how the social "gets under the skin" to affect biology but also how health affects the way we interact with our social world. In this volume, the contribution of Heilmann et al. emphasizes how oral health is shaped by social factors, especially the conditions children experience when they grow up; while the chapter by Taylor-Robinson et al. looks at how the social background of people with cystic fibrosis affects the care they receive and also how the severity of the disease reduces their chances of employment.

The Added Value of the Life Course Perspective to the Analysis of Health

Developed in the social sciences in the 1960s, life course research represents a major shift in the study of human life. It aims at analysing human development throughout the lifespan, considering together processes originally examined separately (Elder 1998; Featherman and Lerner 1985; Sapin et al. 2014). The comprehensive approach of the life course perspective offers important insights with specific relevance for the study of health trajectories, as will be described in this section.

The notion of time is central to the life course perspective. As human development and ageing are life-long processes, research in this domain extends across the successive segments of life or life stages: "different periods across the life course influence phases of biological development, stability or decline" (Ben-Shlomo and Kuh 2002, p. 286). Contrasting but interwoven aspects of time can influence health trajectories, in particular individual ageing and social change. Individual ageing is associated with biological development and decline and with successive social life stages. Research documents 'standard' trajectories and identifies factors associated with deviations from normal paths (non-normative trajectories). In parallel, social change determines specific life conditions since exposure to different risks is time-associated (Wadsworth 1997). Behaviours change over historical time, as for example with smoking patterns: "it is possible to be born into a period of high prevalence of parental smoking and to have lived middle life in a time of much reduced likelihood of smoking" (Wadsworth 1997, p. 864). Patterns of infectious illnesses vary over historical periods of time, as a result of contagion or vaccination. Transformations in medical care and efficacy of treatment also intervene, including the growing capacity to detect diseases earlier in life than before. Changes in policy for example regarding education and in social norms such as those illustrated by the increasing rate of divorce are also time-dependent (Wadsworth 1997). The chapter by Wilmoth et al. in this volume, examining the body mass index trajectories of men who served in the military, offers important insights on the importance of comparing cohorts who lived in distinct historical periods. Therefore the life course perspective promotes analyses that take into account both social and biological opportunities at a specific historical time.

Both structure and agency contribute to an understanding of health inequalities (Abel and Frohlich 2012). The life course perspective also emphasizes the important role that social structures and individual resources play in the development of different trajectories (Elder 1998). It has been noted that, along with structural factors, agency associated with health behaviours account for a part of inequalities in the incidence of diabetes (Kumari et al. 2004; Wikström et al. 2011), obesity (Giskes et al. 2009), functional impairment (Lantz et al. 2001) and poor self-rated health (Joung et al. 1995; Lantz et al. 2001). Life course epidemiology is then interested in how health behaviours and psychosocial resources constitute domains of agency through which individuals influence, positively or negatively, their health over time. In the open debate regarding the origins of disease, studies keep estimating how much individuals influence the development of their own health through their personal resources and behaviours. Modelling trajectories of health behaviours with British cohort data suggested that health behaviours and body mass index could account for almost half of the socioeconomic inequalities in the incidence of type 2 diabetes (Stringhini et al. 2012). Similarly, analyses among young adults concluded that change in psychological resources moderates the evolution of inequalities in distress symptoms: socioeconomic differences increased among respondents having low psychological resources, while these differences remained similar among those with stable or increasing resources (Kiviruusu et al. 2012). Therefore examining the longitudinal influence of agency is likely to contribute to disentangling the effects of different determinants of health. As an illustration, Missinne in this volume analyses the development of health lifestyles, specifically mammogram behaviours, in relationship with respondents' social mobility.

Individuals live in interdependence or in situated networks of relationships. Significant others share similar environmental influences, such as household income, division of domestic tasks, eating patterns or holidays. These elements, referring to the linked lives principle in the life course perspective, are also shaping health behaviours and chronic disease management through mutual influences within the couple, the household or among close friends. Evidence exists that diagnosis of a serious illness and its associated distress impact on both the patients and their spouse (Berg and Upchurch 2007; Booker and Sacker 2012), depression affects one's partner's cognitive functioning (Hinton et al. 2009) and cognitive decline over time is influenced by the spouse (Gerstorf et al. 2009; Gruber-Baldini et al. 1995). The influence of these connections between significant others and individual trajectories remains neglected in empirical research (Bird and Krüger 2005): according to recent reviews, family and health research still focuses on individuals rather than on couples or households as units of analysis (Carr and Springer 2010; Hoppmann and Gerstorf 2009; Pietromonaco et al. 2013). Taking into account individuals' social circumstances needs consideration of their close relationships over time, adding another level of complexity in life course epidemiology analyses.

Family studies and occupational health have contributed to the study of inequalities in health. However, life course epidemiology only recently integrated the family and work lives spheres (Cullati et al. 2014a; Worts et al. 2013). Individuals spend most of their lifetime in these spheres, which (clearly) influence health trajectories. In regard to the work sphere, longitudinal studies show that having secure employment with good working conditions reduces the risks of developing a limiting illness (Bartley et al. 2004); unemployment is associated with higher mortality and morbidity and lower quality of life (Bartley 1994; Booker and Sacker 2013; Flint et al. 2013; McKee-Ryan et al. 2005; Roelfs et al. 2011); and poor psychosocial work environment is a cause of mental disorders (Stansfeld and Candy 2006) and heart disease (Sacker et al. 2001). With regard to the family sphere, it was shown that the family environment not only shapes the life course of individuals but also deeply influences their wellbeing (Uhlenberg and Mueller 2003). Recent research examining the increasing diversity in family structures emphasizes that parenthood and parenting experiences influence wellbeing over life (Umberson et al. 2010). Growing evidence suggests that the accumulation of social roles affects both men's and women's health (Bartley et al. 1999; Bianchi and Milkie 2010). It is known that work-family conflict affects individuals' health (Allen et al. 2000; Eby et al. 2005) and their use of medical drugs (Lallukka et al. 2013), however most of the evidence is based on cross-sectional studies. There is clearly a need to understand better how the intersection of work and family lives imprints into the health trajectories of individuals (Cullati 2014). Indeed individuals experience changing levels of work-family conflict during specific life stages, such as when having young children at home or providing care to older parents (Bianchi and Milkie 2010; Rantanen et al. 2012). Life course epidemiology may thus help identify vulnerable subgroups at specific life stages and inform public policies accordingly.

Research developing at the intersection of social epidemiology and the life course perspective suggests new hypotheses that can help understand how health trajectories are shaped. Looking at social factors (socioeconomic resources, gender roles, changing risks and opportunities), psychological resources (coping mechanisms, resilience and vulnerability), and physiological transformations (ageing, emergence of symptoms, disease, frailty and disability) in a dynamic way clearly opens up promising research questions.

Theoretical Models in Life Course Epidemiology

To formulate hypotheses associating trajectories and transitions, different theoretical models have been discussed in the life course epidemiology literature: the critical (sensitive) period model, the pathway model and the accumulation model (Blane et al. 2007; Graham 2002; Kuh et al. 2003). These models anticipate different patterns and therefore help clarify the mechanisms through which individuals' multiple trajectories interact.

The critical period model assumes that part of the differences in health observed across social groups is explained by exposures occurring in specific periods of development. Deprivation, illness, divorce, risk behaviours (for example smoking, unbalanced diet) are such exposures. Because of their timing, hitting individuals in those critical periods of their life course, these events might lead to irreversible damages or diseases (Ben-Shlomo and Kuh 2002; Marmot and Wadsworth 1997). At first, critical periods have been chiefly related to the biological, cognitive and psychosocial development during foetal life, infancy and childhood. The biological programming hypothesis formulated by David Barker (1997) suggests that poor nutrition during foetal life is associated with increased risk of diseases in adult life. Consequently, authors have suggested that other critical periods for psychosocial and social development may be important for health. Examples include entry into the labour market, leaving the parental home, establishing one's own residence, the transition to parenthood, job insecurity, or exit from the labour market (Bartley et al. 1997). In this volume, the chapter by Johnson et al. dedicated to body size and cardio-metabolic health examines the influences on trajectories of critical periods and transitions, occurring both at the biological and behavioural level. Since social scientists consider that the term "critical period" primarily resonates with biological determinism, they prefer the notion of "sensitive period" (Ben-Shlomo and Kuh 2002; Bornstein 1989; Halfon and Hochstein 2002), or "time associated vulnerability" (Wadsworth 1999). These propose a less deterministic model, where an exposure in a particular period of the life span increases the risk of but does not necessarily result in irreversible damage.

The pathway model hypothesises that the effect of early disadvantage is indirect (Graham 2002). It highlights the different factors, such as lifestyles, educational achievement, social class, health behaviours that can act as mediators between early life social situations and adult health. For example, childhood adversity might restrict educational opportunities which in turn restrict socioeconomic wealth and resources, which in turn influence health behaviours, resulting in poorer health in late life. This model considers that the effect of early life factors on health later in life can be modified to some extent by circumstances occurring at various life stages (Power and Hertzman 1997). The metaphor of the domino aptly summarises the pathway model, also called the "trigger" model.

The accumulation model suggests that life course exposure to adverse environmental and socioeconomic conditions and to health damaging behaviours accumulate over time. Two main fields can be identified: first, the accumulative risk model examines the sum of adverse exposures and risks in the lives of individuals and how these have an increasing influence on health outcomes over time. Second, the cumulative advantage and disadvantage model considers that those with advantaged origins tend to experience subsequent advantageous life course trajectories (O'Rand 1996, 2009), resulting in increasing differences with underprivileged groups over time (Dannefer 2003). This model emphasizes how advantaging or disadvantaging characteristics exert accruing positive or negative influences on health; in contrast, the pathway model emphasizes the paths between the early life advantages or disadvantages and later adult health. The cumulative advantage and disadvantage model, "concerned [...] with questions of fairness in the distribution of opportunities and resources" (Dannefer 2003, p. S327) postulates increasingly diverging patterns in health trajectories.

Variations of these models are also discussed in the present volume. For example Taylor-Robinson et al. make reference to the Diderichsen model identifying four main pathways in the development of health inequalities over the life course, integrating social causation and social selection mechanisms, and Johnson et al. to the developmental origins of health and disease (DOHaD) model. All these models are attractive, but it is also clear that their application is associated with difficulties. One limitation is the absence of theoretical developments addressing the potential reversibility of these processes. Indeed, some life course mechanisms are reversible and should be examined in regard to their negative and positive effects, respectively: for example marriage or divorce can bring either opportunity or adversity in the individual life course (O'Rand 2009); similarly, new employment can bring either better wealth and role enhancement or role overload and life strain. Another problem relates to the fact that even though the empirical testing of these models has increased (Hallqvist et al. 2004; Lynch 2003; Mishra et al. 2009), such findings have rarely been synthesised in systematic reviews (Niedzwiedz et al. 2012; Pollitt et al. 2005). For example we showed that explicit references to the cumulative advantage and disadvantage model remain limited in longitudinal analyses of health trajectories (Cullati et al. 2014b). Different reasons could explain this, including the availability of relevant data (as discussed in the next section) and the difficulty to operationalise in statistical models the assumptions of the theoretical models.

Methodological Considerations in the Study of Health Trajectories

Analysing health trajectories requires repeated measurements. A minimum of two measures is necessary to observe change over time, a minimum of three measures allows description of patterns in trajectories. Longitudinal databases, initiated in the United Kingdom with birth cohorts as early as 1946, are becoming more common. Household panel data available in different countries offer repeated measurements of indicators related to health and social conditions. In a few countries, mostly Scandinavian, unique identification numbers attributed to each citizen allow linkage of data from a range of sources (census, social surveys, medical records...) providing rich information over the individual life span (Blane et al. 2007). Retrospective data, such as collected through life-grid techniques (for example in the SHARE study), also give access to longer periods of time, making possible connections between earlier life events and later health trajectories, but with a risk of information bias.

Investigation of the life course is a progressive research programme that raises new encompassing questions which require the development of new methods, such as large-scale social surveys that include the collection of biomedical data (Blane et al. 2013). However such projects raise ethical issues and public concerns that can impede their developments, as illustrated by the failure of the Swiss Etiological Study of Adjustment and Mental Health (SESAM) (Kummer 2011). Next to challenges associated with work in interdisciplinary teams that bring together social and biological scientists, statistical expertise is required to analyse longitudinal data, adding another layer of complexity. Important questions arise around the empirical analysis of the theoretical models. In this volume, Bell and Jones underline the perils of modelling age, period and cohort effects and propose a theory driven approach to conceptualise these effects. In a chapter combining a methodological discussion and empirical results, Hoekstra and Twisk compare the contributions of latent class growth models and mixed models to the analysis of health trajectories. Ghisletta et al. also examine the advantages and limitations of different statistical models, namely linear mixed-effects models and structural equation models.

While life course epidemiology remains centred on the analysis of quantitative data, we consider that qualitative data are also needed to improve our understanding of health trajectories. Meanings associated with transitions and social hierarchies, expectations of successive cohorts of elderly people ageing in better health conditions are important elements in the complex experience of health. As initiated with work on lay views on health inequalities (Davidson et al. 2006; Popay et al. 1998), data from in-depth individual or collective interviews can inform on mechanisms that relate social and physiological aspects of individual life courses. Qualitative data collected with people suffering from specific conditions are needed to understand their trajectories and their interpretations of biological and social vulnerability.

Policy Implications of Knowledge Gained on Health Trajectories and Transitions

The persistence of health inequalities across contrasting regimes of welfare and health system access is striking (Marmot 2004; Mackenbach 2012). Increasing health inequalities observed in several countries over the last decades (Mackenbach 2012) have been associated with socioeconomic changes but also with the crisis of welfare systems (Bourque and Quesnel-Vallée 2006). This section considers how the life course perspective can contribute to framing public policies that reduce differences in health chances across social categories and generations.

Evidence provided by life course epidemiology can help to identify when measures should intervene in individuals' life span. In the recommendations of the Marmot Review of social determinants and the health divide of the European region (Marmot et al. 2012), adopting a life course perspective is considered as one of the priority areas of action with a focus on children's health: "the highest priority is for countries to ensure a good start in life for every child" (p. 1012). This is expected to contribute to the reduction of health inequalities today, but also in the future by ensuring more health equity across generations, hence addressing the plea of the WHO commission on social determinants of health 'Closing the gap in one generation' (CSDH 2008). The WHO report on life course perspectives on coronary heart disease, stroke and diabetes (Aboderin et al. 2001) also suggested developing policies focused on early life, monitoring growth trajectories of those born into socially or biologically disadvantaged families. This report identified further areas of intervention for later stages of the life span, such as promoting smoking cessation and alcohol reduction programmes among adolescents and adults, and reducing workplace stress among working age adults. In this book, the review by Howe et al. of the evidence on age transitions into obesity during childhood and the degree to which obesity persists over time also discuss how to identify optimal timing for obesity prevention.

The life course perspective emphasizes the need to develop policies that can meet people's needs over the lifespan in their different life spheres. Policies that protect families are expected to have a favourable effect on the health of both parents and children (Bourque and Quesnel-Vallée 2006), especially when policies can address the challenges associated with transitions in family life (birth of children, successive unions, care provided to elderly parents). Policies that protect workers are also likely to have an impact on health trajectories. Analyses of the 2008 crisis showed that employment protection policies mitigated the increased risks of job loss for individuals in poor health in the new economic environment (Reeves et al. 2014). Life course epidemiology further helps to identify vulnerable groups whose needs might require specific measures. For example, a comparison between the United Kingdom and Sweden showed that the Swedish welfare system reduced the poverty and work insecurity of single mothers compared to couple mothers, but that single mothers still reported poorer health status (Whitehead et al. 2000). These results highlight the complex social mechanisms that affect single parenthood and call for policy measures addressing this specific situation. Similarly, Reeves et al. concluded that labour protection policies only have a limited impact on the most vulnerable groups (disabled people, individuals suffering from a chronic disease) during severe recessions, suggesting that next to employment protection, anti-discrimination policies are needed to avoid increasing health inequalities (Reeves et al. 2014).

Accumulating evidence in life course epidemiology emphasizes that health trajectories result from interactions between social and biological processes. Promoting medical care and encouraging healthy behaviours are therefore clearly important domains of action (Braveman et al. 2011; Marmot et al. 2012), but they remain focused on individual determinants of health. Policies across all domains of social life are also called for, to promote healthier environments, at community, national and global levels, in order to limit the impact of threats on health such as the economic crisis, but also climate change (Marmot et al. 2012). Taking into account the social determinants of health in a whole-of-society and life course perspective is expected to contribute to the reduction of health inequalities and to mitigate the intergenerational transmission of risks and disadvantages. On the whole, this will provide economic benefits, but also improve overall quality of life and reinforce social cohesion (Marmot et al. 2012).

State of the Field and Contributions of the Volume

The intersection of social epidemiology and the life course perspective is fairly recent. This volume shows that the field is expanding, with groups developing in different contexts. Infrastructure and resources required for this effort are also extending. These will help to further establish life course research groups, such as the International Centre For Life Course Studies In Society and Health at University College London, the University of Antwerp's Centre for Longitudinal and Life Course Studies (CELLO), and the National Center for Competence in Research LIVES – Overcoming vulnerability over the life course – at the Universities of Lausanne and Geneva. Developments will also be strengthened through the funding of biomedical data collection as part of large-scale social surveys and the promotion of open academic access to these publically funded data. On the academic side, progressive institutionalisation can be observed with the establishment of learned societies, the organization of scientific conferences, work-shops and summer schools. Further efforts should focus on comparisons between countries and international projects. Challenges exist in regard to the integration of interdisciplinary theoretical models and sophisticated statistical analyses, which requires collaborative interdisciplinary work, allowing a mix of skills to pursue the ambitions of life course epidemiology.

This volume brings together nine contributions selected upon propositions received after a wide distribution of the call for papers at the international level. The authors of these contributions represent a range of disciplines and countries, including Switzerland, United States of America, the Netherlands, Belgium, New Zealand and United Kingdom. The chapters combine a mix of reviews, empirical analyses and methodological contributions. They address a range of health topics including obesity, oral health, coronary heart disease, mammogram screening, and cystic fibrosis and take into account different life stages, from childhood to late life. In the absence of clear criteria to structure the presentation of the contributions, we opted for a 'random' order for the first six chapters. The last three contributions have a common focus on methodological and statistical aspects.

The first chapter, *Trajectories and transitions in childhood and adolescent obesity* by Laura Howe, Riz Firestone, Kate Tilling and Debbie Lawlor, offers a review of the evidence regarding trajectories and transitions in childhood and adolescent obesity. The rising prevalence of obesity has turned it into a major public health preoccupation, despite some variations across high-income countries. The chapter shows how adopting a life course perspective improves our understanding of long term consequences of overweight and obesity in early life. Longitudinal analyses provide important insights, assessing how distinct obesity trajectories unfold over time, taking into account the potential persistence of such situations as people age. The authors also discuss how existing data help evaluate the impact of prevention activities and improve their outcome thanks to a better understanding of changes over time.

The second chapter is dedicated to a less visible issue, but of great public health importance, i.e. health related to conditions of the teeth, gums and mouth. In *Oral health over the life course*, Anja Heilmann, Georgios Tsakos and Richard Watt show how these diseases are socially distributed, such differences being accentuated by the high costs associated with their treatment. Oral health is related to general health and affects individuals' quality of life. However, despite its obvious dynamic nature, only limited work examines oral health in a life course perspective. Reviewing the existing literature, the authors emphasize how oral health in adult life is associated with conditions encountered in childhood and how social mobility contributes to distinct trajectories in that domain. Discussing the relevance of the critical period model and the cumulative (dis)advantage model they make suggestions about how this field should pursue its developments.

In *A life course perspective on body size and cardio-metabolic health*, William Johnson, Diana Kuh and Rebecca Hardy are interested in the relationship between birth weight and coronary heart disease. Moving beyond the developmental origins of health and disease (DOHaD) model, the authors propose a lifelong view of the environmental exposures and biological pathways associating body size and cardio-metabolic health. Reviewing the substantial amount of research that has developed over the last 25 years, they describe evidence regarding specific life stages (from gestation to adulthood) and identify three possible trajectories, emphasizing the many factors that can affect the observed associations. They also assess the role of socio-cultural factors and biological pathways and discuss the interactions between these influences, with a focus on transitions, at the biological and social level, that can influence trajectories. They call for the integration of biological and social research in order to understand how to limit the progress of disease in more vulnerable groups.

David Taylor-Robinson, Peter Diggle, Rosalind Smyth and Margaret Whitehead wrote a chapter entitled *Health trajectories in people with cystic fibrosis in the UK: exploring the effect of social deprivation*. They analyse the influence of social factors on the trajectories of these people. Considering that there are no socioeconomic differences in the incidence of cystic fibrosis since it has a genetic origin, they analyse the trajectories of those affected and identified during childhood to reveal social patterns in the outcomes associated with cystic fibrosis. The contribution brings together results from longitudinal registry studies that examine the impact of social deprivation on clinical outcomes, health care use and employment opportunities. The findings show social deprivation differences in clinical outcomes, with individuals living in more affluent areas having better lung function and less pseudomonas aeruginosa (the most common pathogen causing chronic infection in those with cystic fibrosis) chronic colonisation. Treatments differ across social groups and inequalities grow after the transition to adult care.

Employment chances vary along social resources, disease severity and time spent in hospital. Observing that inequalities start early in the trajectories of those diagnosed with cystic fibrosis, the contribution confirms the importance of action taken at the beginning of life and supports the development of public health policies focused on early life experiences. Implications of the findings for health care systems and for clinicians are also discussed.

The next chapter, *Moving towards a better understanding of socioeconomic inequalities in preventive health care use: a life course perspective* by Sarah Missinne, examines how the life course perspective can also contribute to the study of socioeconomic factors in preventive behaviours. Pursuing different recent theoretical developments in medical sociology that take into account a longer-term view of individual health, she analyses mammography screening in the light of the five principles of the life course perspective. Including the life-span development principle helps to clarify how healthy lifestyles are adopted and maintained. The timing principle allows analyses of regularity and timeliness in preventive health care. Socialization contexts affect health-related lifestyles, illustrating the structure-agency debate. Comparisons across different European countries show the importance of policy contexts. And finally her analyses confirm the importance of the linked lives principle with the role played by significant others in the use of preventive measures.

In *Inter-Cohort Variation in the Consequences of U.S. Military Service on Men's Body Mass Index Trajectories in Mid- to Late-Life*, Janet Wilmoth, Andrew London and Christine Himes are also interested in obesity as a particularly important public health preoccupation in the United States. Their analysis compares trajectories of veterans who served in the army with those of men of mid- to-late life, including different successive cohorts of men born during the first half of the twentieth century. Different mechanisms affecting veterans' health are discussed, including positive factors such as intense physical training and fitness required to be in the army and negative factors such as training accidents or stressors related to separation from family and work. Analyses controlling for birth cohort, early-life factors and mid- to late-life influences indicate that veterans are marginally heavier than their civil counterparts. The study demonstrates a large secular effect in increasing weight among successive cohorts and a small but consistent intra-cohort effect.

The volume then presents three papers addressing methodological issues in the analyses of health trajectories and transitions, in particular specific issues associated with longitudinal data. In *Linear mixed-effects and latent curve models for longitudinal life course analyses,* Paolo Ghisletta, Olivier Renaud, Nadège Jacot and Delphine Courvoisier emphasize how longitudinal data cannot be analysed with standard statistical models since these data, collected with the same individuals, are inherently dependent. They present linear mixed-effects models and structural equation models, more appropriate for quantitative longitudinal data since they explicitly define parameters related to both stability and change processes. Furthermore, these models present the advantage that they allow analysis of the interactions between individuals and their context, considering that these characteristics can be stable or can vary over time. The authors further discuss the advantages of these models and their recent developments, such as dealing with incomplete data, multivariate specifications, comparisons of groups, and latent class analyses that uncover group membership through statistical analyses. Illustrations for these different arguments are provided with analyses conducted with data of the Swiss Household Panel.

Trynke Hoekstra and Jos Twisk also highlight difficulties associated with repeated observations in longitudinal data. As indicated by its title, *The analysis of individual health trajectories across the life course: Latent class growth models versus mixed models,* their contribution is focused on two types of models that allow the integration of successive stages in the life course trajectory. The authors discuss the specificities of both statistical models, including extensions that allow measuring possible heterogeneity in health trajectories. They illustrate their points by analyses of body mass index trajectories with data of the Amsterdam Growth and Health Study cohort, first started in 1974 with teenagers.

Last but not least, the contribution of Andrew Bell and Kelvyn Jones considers age, period and cohort effects. The chapter *Age, period and cohort processes in longitudinal and life course analysis: a multilevel perspective* envisions these different effects as sources of health-related change, combining biological and social factors. Naive life course approaches can produce misleading results if these different effects – age, period and cohort (APC) – are not carefully examined to understand if they could be generating mathematical confounding. Using the example of obesity, the authors show the limits of some of the currently used APC models and they offer an extension that aims at modelling these different effects in a robust and explicit way. In their case, illustrations of their arguments are based on analyses of the British Household Panel Survey.

This volume has been made possible by the commitment of the authors to prepare and revise their chapters. In fact, we also want to emphasize the important contribution of the reviewers we have sollicited over the preparation of this book. We want to warmly thank: Thomas Abel, Mel Bartley, Patrick Bodenmann, Stefano Cavalli, Paul Clarke, Laurie Corna, Angela Donkin, Jacques-Antoine Gauthier, Francesco Giudici, Anne McMunn, Scott Montgomery, Sam Norton, France Weaver and Dick Wiggins, for their thorough reviews. We are also grateful to the editors of the collection, Laura Bernardi, Dario Spini and Michel Oris, for their support in the preparation of this volume. Generous funding received from the NCCR LIVES – Overcoming vulnerability over the life course – has made this publication possible, especially its open access online edition.

We hope this volume will be of interest for researchers working in different domains, in particular health and social sciences, and reinforce the attention to be paid to the unfolding of individuals' health histories. Considering that these result from complex interactive effects associating transitions within individuals' bodies and lives with changes in the broader social environment, the contributions offer theoretical insights, methodological developments and empirical results whose policy implications should be acknowledged by those who can impact governmental measures.

References

Abel, T., & Frohlich, K. L. (2012). Capitals and capabilities: Linking structure and agency to reduce health inequalities. *Social Science & Medicine, 74*(2), 236–244. doi:10.1016/j.socscimed.2011.10.028.

Aboderin, I., Kalache, A., Ben-Shlomo, Y., Lynch, J. W., Yajnik, C. S., Kuh, D., & Yach, D. (2001). *Life course perspectives on coronary heart disease, stroke and diabetes: Key issues and implications for policy and research*. Geneva: World Health Organization.

Allen, T. D., Herst, D. E. L., Bruck, C. S., & Sutton, M. (2000). Consequences associated with work-to-family conflict: A review and agenda for future research. *Journal of Occupational Health Psychology, 5*(2), 278–308. doi:10.1037/1076-8998.5.2.278.

Anderson, N. B. (1998). Levels of analysis in health science: A framework for integrating sociobehavioral and biomedical research. *Annals of the New York Academy of Sciences, 840*(1), 563–576. doi:10.1111/j.1749-6632.1998.tb09595.x.

Barker, D. J. P. (1997). Maternal nutrition, fetal nutrition, and disease in later life. *Nutrition, 13*(9), 807–813. doi:10.1016/s0899-9007(97)00193-7.

Bartley, M. (1994). Unemployment and ill health: Understanding the relationship. *Journal of Epidemiology and Community Health, 48*(4), 333–337. doi:10.1136/jech.48.4.333.

Bartley, M., Blane, D., & Montgomery, S. (1997). Health and the life course: Why safety nets matter. *BMJ, 314*(7088), 1194–1196.

Bartley, M., Sacker, A., Firth, D., & Fitzpatrick, R. (1999). Social position, social roles and women's health in England: Changing relationships 1984–1993. *Social Science & Medicine, 48*(1), 99–115. doi:10.1016/S0277-9536(98)00293-7.

Bartley, M., Sacker, A., & Clarke, P. (2004). Employment status, employment conditions, and limiting illness: Prospective evidence from the British household panel survey 1991–2001. *Journal of Epidemiology and Community Health, 58*(6), 501–506. doi:10.1136/jech.2003.009878.

Ben-Shlomo, Y., & Kuh, D. (2002). A life course approach to chronic disease epidemiology: Conceptual models, empirical challenges and interdisciplinary perspectives. *International Journal of Epidemiology, 31*(2), 285–293. doi:10.1093/ije/31.2.285.

Berg, C. A., & Upchurch, R. (2007). A developmental-contextual model of couples coping with chronic illness across the adult life span. *Psychological Bulletin, 133*(6), 920–954. doi:10.1037/0033-2909.133.6.920.

Bianchi, S. M., & Milkie, M. A. (2010). Work and family research in the first decade of the 21st century. *Journal of Marriage and Family, 72*(3), 705–725. doi:10.1111/j.1741-3737.2010.00726.x.

Bird, K., & Krüger, H. (2005). The secret of transitions: The interplay of complexity and reduction in life course analysis. In R. Levy, P. Ghisletta, J.-M. Le Goff, D. Spini, & E. Widmer (Eds.), *Towards an interdisciplinary perspective on the life course* (Advances in life course research, Vol. 10, pp. 173–194). Amsterdam: Elsevier.

Blane, D., Netuveli, G., & Stone, J. (2007). The development of life course epidemiology. *Revue d'Épidémiologie et de Santé Publique, 55*(1), 31–38. doi:10.1016/j.respe.2006.12.004.

Blane, D., Kelly-Irving, M., d'Errico, A., Bartley, M., & Montgomery, S. (2013). Social-biological transitions: How does the social become biological? *Longitudinal and Life Course Studies, 4*(2), 136–146. doi:10.14301/llcs.v4i2.236.

Booker, C. L., & Sacker, A. (2012). Limiting long-term illness and subjective well-being in families. *Longitudinal and Life Course Studies, 3*(1), 41–65. doi:10.14301/llcs.v3i1.160.

Booker, C. L., & Sacker, A. (2013). Labour force sequences, unemployment spells and their effect on subjective well-being set points. *Longitudinal and Life Course Studies, 4*(2), 88–104. doi:10.14301/llcs.v4i2.239.

Bornstein, M. H. (1989). Sensitive periods in development: Structural characteristics and causal interpretations. *Psychological Bulletin, 105*(2), 179–197. doi:10.1037/0033-2909.105.2.179.

Bourque, M., & Quesnel-Vallée, A. (2006). Politiques sociales: Un enjeu de santé publique? *Lien social et Politiques, 55*, 45–52.

Braveman, P. A., Egerter, S. A., & Mockenhaupt, R. E. (2011). Broadening the focus. The need to address the social determinants of health. *American Journal of Preventive Medicine, 40*(1), S4–S18. doi:10.1016/j.amepre.2010.10.002.

Carr, D., & Springer, K. W. (2010). Advances in families and health research in the 21st century. *Journal of Marriage and Family, 72*(3), 743–761. doi:10.1111/j.1741-3737.2010.00728.x.

Colerick Clipp, E., Pavalko, E. K., & Elder, G. H. (1992). Trajectories of health: In concept and empirical pattern. *Behavior, Health, & Aging, 2*(3), 159–179.

CSDH. (2008). *Closing the gap in a generation: Health equity through action on the social determinants of health. Final Report of the Commission on Social Determinants of Health.* Geneva: World Health Organization.

Cullati, S. (2014). The influence of work-family conflict trajectories on self-rated health trajectories in Switzerland: A life course approach. *Social Science & Medicine, 113*, 23–33. doi:10.1016/j.socscimed.2014.04.030.

Cullati, S., Courvoisier, D. S., & Burton-Jeangros, C. (2014a). Mental health trajectories and their embeddedness in work and family circumstances: A latent state-trait approach to life-course trajectories. *Sociology of Health & Illness, 36*(7), 1077–1094. doi:10.1111/1467-9566.12156.

Cullati, S., Rousseaux, E., Gabadinho, A., Courvoisier, D. S., & Burton-Jeangros, C. (2014b). Factors of change and cumulative factors in self-rated health trajectories: A systematic review. *Advances in Life Course Research, 19*, 14–27. doi:10.1016/j.alcr.2013.11.002.

Dannefer, D. (2003). Cumulative advantage/disadvantage and the life course: Cross-fertilizing age and social science theory. *Journals of Gerontology. Series B, Psychological Sciences and Social Sciences, 58*(6), 327–337. doi:10.1093/geronb/58.6.S327.

Davidson, R., Kitzinger, J., & Hunt, K. (2006). The wealthy get healthy, the poor get poorly? Lay perceptions of health inequalities. *Social Science & Medicine, 62*(9), 2171–2182. doi:10.1016/j.socscimed.2005.10.010.

Eby, L. T., Casper, W. J., Lockwood, A., Bordeaux, C., & Brinley, A. (2005). Work and family research in IO/OB: Content analysis and review of the literature (1980–2002). *Journal of Vocational Behavior, 66*(1), 124–197. doi:10.1016/j.jvb.2003.11.003.

Elder, G. H., Jr. (1998). The life course as developmental theory. *Child Development, 69*(1), 1–12. doi:10.1111/j.1467-8624.1998.tb06128.x.

Featherman, D. L., & Lerner, R. M. (1985). Ontogenesis and sociogenesis: Problematics for theory and research about development and socialization across the lifespan. *American Sociological Review, 50*(5), 659–676. doi:10.2307/2095380.

Flint, E., Bartley, M., Shelton, N., & Sacker, A. (2013). Do labour market status transitions predict changes in psychological well-being? *Journal of Epidemiology and Community Health, 67*(9), 796–802. doi:10.1136/jech-2013-202425.

Gerstorf, D., Hoppmann, C. A., Kadlec, K. M., & McArdle, J. J. (2009). Memory and depressive symptoms are dynamically linked among married couples: Longitudinal evidence from the AHEAD study. *Developmental Psychology, 45*(6), 1595–1610. doi:10.1037/a0016346.

Giskes, K., Avendano, M., Brug, J., & Kunst, A. E. (2009). A systematic review of studies on socioeconomic inequalities in dietary intakes associated with weight gain and overweight/obesity conducted among European adults. *Obesity Reviews, 11*(6), 413–429.

Glass, T. A., & McAtee, M. J. (2006). Behavioral science at the crossroads in public health: Extending horizons, envisioning the future. *Social Science & Medicine, 62*(7), 1650–1671. doi:10.1016/j.socscimed.2005.08.044.

Graham, H. (2002). Building an inter-disciplinary science of health inequalities: The example of lifecourse research. *Social Science & Medicine, 55*(11), 2005–2016. doi:10.1016/S0277-9536(01)00343-4.

Gruber-Baldini, A. L., Schaie, K. W., & Willis, S. L. (1995). Similarity in married couples: A longitudinal study of mental abilities and rigidity-flexibility. [Research Support, U.S. Gov't, P.H.S.]. *Journal of Personality and Social Psychology, 69*(1), 191–203. doi:10.1037/0022-3514.69.1.191.

Halfon, N., & Hochstein, M. (2002). Life course health development: An integrated framework for developing health, policy, and research. *The Milbank Quarterly, 80*(3), 433–479. doi:10.1111/1468-0009.00019.

Hallqvist, J., Lynch, J., Bartley, M., Lang, T., & Blane, D. (2004). Can we disentangle life course processes of accumulation, critical period and social mobility? An analysis of disadvantaged socio-economic positions and myocardial infarction in the Stockholm Heart Epidemiology Program. *Social Science & Medicine, 58*(8), 1555–1562. doi:10.1016/S0277-9536(03)00344-7.

Hinton, L., Hagar, Y., West, N., Gonzalez, H. M., Mungas, D., Beckett, L., et al. (2009). Longitudinal influences of partner depression on cognitive functioning in Latino spousal pairs. *Dementia and Geriatric Cognitive Disorders, 27*(6), 491–500. doi:10.1159/000218113.

Hoppmann, C., & Gerstorf, D. (2009). Spousal interrelations in old age – a mini-review. *Gerontology, 55*(4), 449. doi:10.1159/000211948.

Huber, M., Knottnerus, J. A., Green, L., van der Horst, H., Jadad, A. R., Kromhout, D., et al. (2011). How should we define health? *BMJ, 343*. doi:10.1136/bmj.d4163.

Joung, I. M., Stronks, K., van de Mheen, H., & Mackenbach, J. P. (1995). Health behaviours explain part of the differences in self reported health associated with partner/marital status in The Netherlands. *Journal of Epidemiology and Community Health, 49*(5), 482–488. doi:10.1136/jech.49.5.482.

Kiviruusu, O., Huurre, T., Haukkala, A., & Aro, H. (2012). Changes in psychological resources moderate the effect of socioeconomic status on distress symptoms: A 10-year follow-up among young adults. *Health Psychology: Official Journal of the Division of Health Psychology, American Psychological* Association. doi:10.1037/a0029291.

Kuh, D. J. L., & Ben-Shlomo, Y. (2004). *A life course approach to chronic disease epidemiology.* New York: Oxford University Press.

Kuh, D. J. L., Ben-Shlomo, Y., Lynch, J., Hallqvist, J., & Power, C. (2003). Life course epidemiology. *Journal of Epidemiology and Community Health, 57*(10), 778–783. doi:10.1136/jech.57.10.778.

Kumari, M., Head, J., & Marmot, M. G. (2004). Prospective study of social and other risk factors for incidence of type 2 diabetes in the Whitehall II study. *Archives of Internal Medicine, 164*(17), 1873–1880. doi:10.1001/archinte.164.17.1873.

Kummer, H. (2011). The Swiss Etiological Study of Adjustment and Mental Health (SESAM). Anatomy of failure of a research project. *Pipette, 1*, 9–13.

Lallukka, T., Arber, S., Laaksonen, M., Lahelma, E., Partonen, T., & Rahkonen, O. (2013). Work-family conflicts and subsequent sleep medication among women and men: A longitudinal registry linkage study. *Social Science & Medicine, 79*, 66–75. doi:10.1016/j.socscimed.2012.05.011.

Lantz, P. M., Lynch, J. W., House, J. S., Lepkowski, J. M., Mero, R. P., Musick, M. A., et al. (2001). Socioeconomic disparities in health change in a longitudinal study of US adults: The role of health-risk behaviors. *Social Science & Medicine, 53*(1), 29–40. doi:10.1016/S0277-9536(00)00319-1.

Lynch, S. M. (2003). Cohort and life-course patterns in the relationship between education and health: A hierarchical approach. *Demography, 40*(2), 309–331. doi:10.1353/dem.2003.0016.

Mackenbach, J. P. (2012). The persistence of health inequalities in modern welfare states: The explanation of a paradox. *Social Science & Medicine, 75*(4), 761–769.

Marmot, M. (2004). *The status syndrome. How social status affects our health and longevity.* New York: Owl Books.

Marmot, M. G., & Wadsworth, M. E. J. (1997). Fetal and early childhood environment: Long-term health implications. *British Medical Bulletin, 53*(1), 3–9.

Marmot, M., Allen, J., Bell, R., Bloomer, E., & Goldblatt, P. (2012). WHO European review of social determinants of health and the health divide. *The Lancet, 380*(9846), 1011–1029.

McKee-Ryan, F., Song, Z., Wanberg, C. R., & Kinicki, A. J. (2005). Psychological and physical well-being during unemployment: A meta-analytic study. *Journal of Applied Psychology, 90*(1), 53–76. doi:10.1037/0021-9010.90.1.53.

Mishra, G. D., Nitsch, D., Black, S., De Stavola, B., Kuh, D., & Hardy, R. (2009). A structured approach to modelling the effects of binary exposure variables over the life course. *International Journal of Epidemiology, 38*(2), 528–537. doi:10.1093/ije/dyn229.

Niedzwiedz, C. L., Katikireddi, S. V., Pell, J. P., & Mitchell, R. (2012). Life course socio-economic position and quality of life in adulthood: A systematic review of life course models. *BMC Public Health, 12*(1), 628. doi:10.1186/1471-2458-12-628.

O'Rand, A. M. (1996). The precious and the precocious: Understanding cumulative disadvantage and cumulative advantage over the life course. *The Gerontologist, 36*(2), 230–238. doi:10.1093/geront/36.2.230.

O'Rand, A. M. (2009). Cumulative processes in the life course. In G. H. Elder & J. Z. Giele (Eds.), *The craft of life course research* (pp. 121–140). New York: Guilford.

Pietromonaco, P. R., Uchino, B., & Dunkel Schetter, C. (2013). Close relationship processes and health: Implications of attachment theory for health and disease. *Health Psychology, 32*(5), 499–513. doi:10.1037/a0029349.

Pollitt, R., Rose, K., & Kaufman, J. (2005). Evaluating the evidence for models of life course socioeconomic factors and cardiovascular outcomes: A systematic review. *BMC Public Health, 5*(1), 7. doi:10.1186%2F1471-2458-5-7.

Popay, J., Williams, G., Thomas, C., & Gatrell, T. (1998). Theorising inequalities in health: The place of lay knowledge. *Sociology of Health & Illness, 20*(5), 619–644. doi:10.1111/1467-9566.00122.

Power, C., & Hertzman, C, (1997). Social and biological pathways linking early life and adult disease. *British Medical Bulletin, 53*(1), 210–221.

Rantanen, J., Kinnunen, U., Pulkkinen, L., & Kokko, K. (2012). Developmental trajectories of work–family conflict for Finnish workers in midlife. *Journal of Occupational Health Psychology, 17*(3), 290–303. doi:10.1037/a0028153.

Reeves, A., Karanikolos, M., Mackenbach, J., McKee, M., & Stuckler, D. (2014). Do employment protection policies reduce the relative disadvantage in the labour market experienced by unhealthy people? A natural experiment created by the Great Recession in Europe. *Social Science & Medicine, 121*, 98–108.

Roelfs, D. J., Shor, E., Davidson, K. W., & Schwartz, J. E. (2011). Losing life and livelihood: A systematic review and meta-analysis of unemployment and all-cause mortality. *Social Science & Medicine, 72*(6), 840–854. doi:10.1016/j.socscimed.2011.01.005.

Sacker, A., Bartley, M., Frith, D., Fitzpatrick, R., & Marmot, M. G. (2001). The relationship between job strain and coronary heart disease: Evidence from an English sample of the working male population. *Psychological Medicine, 31*(02), 279–290. doi:10.1017/S0033291701003270.

Sapin, M., Spini, D., & Widmer, E. (2014). *Les parcours de vie. De l'adolescence au grand âge* (coll. Le savoir suisse). Lausanne: Presses polytechniques et universitaires romandes.

Stansfeld, S., & Candy, B. (2006). Psychosocial work environment and mental health – A meta-analytic review. *Scandinavian Journal of Work, Environment & Health, 32*(6), 443–462. doi:10.5271/sjweh.1050.

Stringhini, S., Tabak, A. G., Akbaraly, T. N., Sabia, S., Shipley, M. J., Marmot, M. G., et al. (2012). Contribution of modifiable risk factors to social inequalities in type 2 diabetes: Prospective Whitehall II cohort study. *BMJ, 345.* doi:10.1136/bmj.e5452.

Uhlenberg, P., & Mueller, M. (2003). Family context and individual well-being. Patterns and mechanisms in life course perspective. In J. T. Mortimer & M. J. Shanahan (Eds.), *Handbook of the life course* (Handbooks of sociology and social research 2003rd ed., pp. 123–148). New York: Kluwer/Plenum.

Umberson, D., Pudrovska, T., & Reczek, C. (2010). Parenthood, childlessness, and well-being: A life course perspective. *Journal of Marriage and Family, 72*(3), 612–629.

Wadsworth, M. E. J. (1997). Health inequalities in the life course perspective. *Social Science & Medicine, 44*(6), 859–869. doi:10.1016/S0277-9536(96)00187-6.

Wadsworth, M. E. J. (1999). Early life. In M. Marmot & R. G. Wilkinson (Eds.), *Social determinants of health* (pp. 44–63). Oxford: Oxford University Press.

Whitehead, M., Burström, B., & Diderichsen, F. (2000). Social policies and the pathways to inequalities in health: A comparative analysis of lone mothers in Britain and Sweden. *Social Science and Medicine, 50*(2), 255–270.

WHO. (1946). Preamble to the Constitution of the World Health Organization as adopted by the international health conference, New York, 19–22 June 1946. http://www.who.int/about/definition/en/print.html

Wikström, K., Lindström, J., Tuomilehto, J., Saaristo, T. E., Korpi-Hyövälti, E., Oksa, H., et al. (2011). Socio-economic differences in dysglycemia and lifestyle-related risk factors in the Finnish middle-aged population. *The European Journal of Public Health, 21*(6), 768–774. doi:10.1093/eurpub/ckq164.

Wilkinson, R. G. (1996). *Unhealthy societies: The afflictions of inequality*. London: Routledge.

Worts, D., Sacker, A., McMunn, A., & McDonough, P. (2013). Individualization, opportunity and jeopardy in American women's work and family lives: A multi-state sequence analysis. *Advances in Life Course Research, 18*(4), 296–318. doi:10.1016/j.alcr.2013.09.003.

Chapter 2
Trajectories and Transitions in Childhood and Adolescent Obesity

Laura D. Howe, Riz Firestone, Kate Tilling, and Debbie A. Lawlor

Introduction

The last few decades have seen a dramatic rise in the prevalence of overweight and obesity in most high-income countries. This rise has been seen across all ages, even in very young children (Wang and Lobstein 2006). Obesity is now recognised as one of the most important public health concerns of our time (Dietz 2004), and places a considerable burden on healthcare systems; the cost of obesity to the UK economy was estimated in 2007 to be £15.38 billion per year, including £4.2 billion in costs to the National Health Service (Public Health England 2014). Although recent evidence suggests that the increase in childhood obesity may be abating in some countries (Han et al. 2010), it is too soon to be certain that the flattening of the epidemic will continue, and there is no evidence of a decline in the currently high levels. There is wide variation in the prevalence of childhood overweight between European countries (Fig. 2.1). This variability does not notably follow patterns of geographic area, country wealth or political system and suggests that there is potential for the lowest levels to be seen across the whole of Europe. Being overweight or obese as a child is associated with both short- and long-term health risks, particularly for cardiovascular health (Owen et al. 2009; Friedemann

L.D. Howe (✉) • K. Tilling • D.A. Lawlor
MRC Integrative Epidemiology Unit, University of Bristol, Bristol, UK

School of Social and Community Medicine, University of Bristol, Bristol, UK
e-mail: laura.howe@bristol.ac.uk

R. Firestone
Centre for Public Health Research, Massey University, Wellington, New Zealand

© The Author(s) 2015
C. Burton-Jeangros et al. (eds.), *A Life Course Perspective on Health Trajectories and Transitions*, Life Course Research and Social Policies 4,
DOI 10.1007/978-3-319-20484-0_2

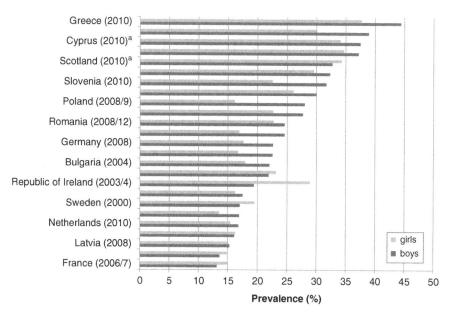

Fig. 2.1 Country-level prevalence of overweight/obesity in children in the European Union Prevalence is shown separately for males (*dark grey*) and females (*light grey*) for countries in the European Union with measured heights and weights, ordered according to prevalence. Data for this figure were obtained from the World Obesity Federation website: http://www.worldobesity.org/site_media/library/resource_images/Child_EU_March_2014_WO.pdf (last accessed 13th March 2014). LD Howe accepts responsibility for accurately converting the data into the above figure [a]Childhood overweight/obesity defined by national reference chart percentiles; for all other countries the International Obesity Task Force (IOTF) criteria were used

et al. 2012) and type two diabetes (Hannon et al. 2005), but also for mental health (Russell-Mayhew et al. 2012) and social outcomes such as educational attainment (von Hinke Kessler Scholder et al. 2012).

A life course perspective can increase our understanding of childhood obesity. There is now strong evidence that pre-natal and early-life factors are involved in the development of childhood obesity (Parsons et al. 1999; Warrington et al. 2013; Howe et al. 2011, 2012; Fairley et al. 2013), and that obesity often begins early in life (Kipping et al. 2008; Reilly and Wilson 2006). Furthermore, despite some interventions with established effectiveness (Picot et al. 2009; Loveman et al. 2011; Ara et al. 2012), adult obesity has proved very difficult to treat (Livhits et al. 2012; Loveman et al. 2011), emphasising the need for early preventative intervention. Utilising longitudinal data from cohort studies enables the study of the dynamic patterns of adiposity development across the life course, and may help to inform the development of intervention strategies. For example, understanding the ages at which obesity tends to develop within children and the degree to which transitions in obesity status occur within children and between childhood and adulthood can provide information about the most appropriate ages for preventative interventions, and the likely population benefits of policies. Life course studies can also yield information about whether distinct trajectories of obesity development have different impacts on later health, and the ways in which the determinants of obesity alter the patterns of adiposity trajectories.

In this chapter, we review evidence from observational studies (i.e. not including data from follow-up studies of interventions) to meet our aims of (i) describing the evidence on the ages at which obesity develops in contemporary cohorts of children and adolescents, (ii) describing the evidence on the persistence (stability, or tracking) of childhood overweight and obesity, and (iii) discussing the added aetiological insight that can be achieved from longitudinal life course studies of childhood overweight and obesity as compared with cross-sectional studies. We conclude by reflecting on the importance of a life course perspective in studies of childhood obesity, and discussing future directions for life course studies in this area.

When Do Children Become Overweight or Obese?

A vast number of studies have documented the prevalence of childhood obesity. In contrast, relatively little research has focused on the *incidence* of obesity during childhood and adolescence. Susceptibility to becoming overweight or obese is likely to vary across the life course due to changing biological, social and behavioural influences. Understanding when in the life course the highest periods of incidence occur is extremely important, since it influences the likely effectiveness of preventative intervention studies targeted at different age groups. In this section of the chapter we will review the evidence on when overweight and obese children became overweight or obese, and discuss the implications of this body of evidence for the optimal timing of obesity prevention interventions.

One British study that generated an enormous amount of media interest was analysis of the EarlyBird cohort by Gardner et al. (2009). This study examined weight gain (defined as an increase in weight z-score [z-scores are age- and sex-standardised measurements, so an increase in weight z-score means an increase in weight given what would be expected from a child's age and sex]) between birth, five years, and nine years in a cohort of 233 children from the south-west of England. The results showed that weight z-scores (using UK 1990 reference data) increased substantially from birth to five years – mean weight z-scores at birth were 0.02 for males and 0.32 for females (i.e. females were considerably heavier at birth than the average birth weight for females in the 1990 reference dataset, but males were similar at birth to the 1990 reference data), increasing to 0.28 at 0.61 at five years for males and females respectively (i.e. both males and females gained more weight between birth and five years than the average pattern of weight gain in the 1990 reference dataset). From five years to nine years there was a much smaller increase in weight z-scores – 0.28 to 0.39 in males and 0.61 to 0.64 in females. The authors reported strong correlations between weight z-score at ages five and nine; 0.89 in males and 0.84 in females, both P < 0.001. The widely-publicised interpretation of these results was that the preschool period was critical in the development of excess weight gain. The implication of this conclusion is that obesity prevention interventions should focus primarily on preschool children. The authors state that "If excess weight gain were prevented during the preschool age, our data imply that a healthier weight might be maintained thereafter". They also suggest that potential risk factors in school-aged children should be de-emphasised, stating "given the pattern of weight gain reported here, the contribution to childhood obesity by computers, school meals, (lack of) sports clubs, (absence of) school playing fields, and the 'school-run' (all of which are vilified regularly by the media) might be questioned". This analysis of the EarlyBird study, however, included only 233 children with weight as the only measure of adiposity, and measurements at just three ages – birth, five and nine years (Gardner et al. 2009).

In response to the EarlyBird study, Hughes et al. conducted similar analyses in the Avon Longitudinal Study of Parents and Children (ALSPAC) (Hughes et al. 2011b). In this cohort, repeated measurements of weight and height were available from birth to age 15 years for 625 children. The authors conducted similar analyses to Gardner et al. (2009), but made use of z-scores for both body mass index (BMI) and weight, rather than relying only on weight as in the EarlyBird publication. In contrast to the findings of Gardner et al., Hughes et al. reported that mean weight and BMI z-scores increased steadily as the children got older, with the changes being most marked after school entry age (age five years). For example, the mean z-scores for weight in study participants were 0.12 at birth, 0.22 at 1 year, 0.20 at 3 years, 0.18 at 5 years, 0.22 at 7 years, 0.37 at 9 years, 0.54 at 11 years, 0.51 at 13 years, and 0.48 at 15 years. The change in z-scores between birth and five years was not statistically significant, whereas the change in weight z-scores between five and nine years was statistically significant; mean difference in males was 0.26, P < 0.001 and in females was 0.10, P < 0.001. A similar pattern was seen for BMI z-scores, with no statistical evidence of a difference in the rate of change in z-scores when comparing the periods between one and five years or five and nine years (Hughes et al. 2011b). Thus these results do not corroborate the findings of Gardner et al., and instead suggest that weight status is not set by the time of school entry. Considerable excess weight gain (defined by increases in weight and BMI z-scores) was observed in mid-childhood in this cohort. This casts doubt on the idea that obesity prevention initiatives should be focused on preschool children, and instead implies that policies should target children of all ages.

Differences between the analysis of ALSPAC by Hughes et al. and the EarlyBird paper include a much larger sample size, use of both weight and BMI to define adiposity, and analysis of a greater period of childhood – birth to 15 years in ALSPAC, with detailed data across the first five years, in contrast to three measures at birth, five and nine years in the EarlyBird study. Other factors may also contribute to the different findings, including differences in birth years (1992 in ALSPAC, 1995 in EarlyBird), sociodemographic and geographical factors. Further analysis of the ALSPAC data using alternative methodology also suggests that weight status is not set at school entry. Using data on more than 4,000 children, Hughes et al.

(2011a) found a five-year incidence of obesity (defined as BMI above the 95th centile according to the UK 1990 reference, i.e. using a threshold to define obesity as opposed to using z-scores as a continuous variable in the previous paper) of 5 % between ages seven and 11 years. This was higher than the incidence observed between ages 11 and 15 years (1.4 %). In the subset of the cohort for whom data was available before age seven (N = 549), the incidence of obesity was 5.1 % between three and seven years, 6.7 % between seven and 11 years, and 1.6 % between 11 and 15 years (Hughes et al. 2011a). These data do not support the hypothesis that most excess weight gain occurs before age five years; rather they suggest that mid-childhood is a period during which young people are particularly susceptible to develop obesity.

Other studies have also provided evidence for excess weight gain or obesity development in school-aged children. Most of these studies do not have adiposity data from before age five, and so cannot assess changes in weight or BMI z-scores between birth and school entry, but the studies can provide evidence about the degree of weight gain and obesity development during mid- and late-childhood. In one study in the USA, 5,940 children were assessed in Kindergarten (mean age 5.7 years) and then monitored over the next nine years (Datar et al. 2011). At the start of the study, almost 40 % of the children had a BMI above the 75th centile according to Center for Disease Control (CDC) growth charts. This percentage increased by 5.8 % in the first three years of the study, with a mean change in BMI z-scores of 3.3. These first three years from age 5.7 years were the period with the greatest increases in BMI. In this study there was little further increase in BMI after approximately age 13 years. The authors noted that the increases in mean BMI z-score as the children got older were to a large extent driven by increases in obesity (defined as BMI above the 95th centile); obesity prevalence increased by almost 50 % in the first four years – from 11.9 % in Kindergarten to 17.6 % in the third grade, remaining fairly stable after this age. It is worth noting, however, that these figures do demonstrate that the majority of obese children were already obese at entry into Kindergarten.

Further evidence of excess weight gain during childhood comes from analyses of the US National Health and Nutrition Examination Surveys (NHANES) (Flegal and Troiano 2000). In these (cross-sectional) studies, obesity prevalence was found to be higher among 9–11 year olds compared with six to eight year olds, suggesting that some children gain excessive weight and become obese during mid-childhood. These analyses, however, found that there was little difference in the obesity prevalence comparing nine to 11 year olds with older adolescents up to age 17 years (Flegal and Troiano 2000; Ogden et al. 2010).

Support for limited change in obesity prevalence during adolescence (i.e. after approximately age 11 years) is also provided by analysis of the ALSPAC data, which showed only a 1.4 % incidence of obesity between ages 11 and 15 years (Hughes et al. 2011a), and by several other studies. Wardle et al. reported that persistent obesity was generally established before age 11 (Wardle et al. 2006). In analyses of data from 5,863 English school children, the authors reported that obesity prevalence at entry to the study (age 11–12 years) was almost 25 %. During five years of follow-up, the obesity prevalence did rise – but in the majority of cases this was because of overweight children becoming obese; the proportion of children in the healthy BMI category remained stable. Little evidence was found of new cases of overweight or obesity emerging between ages 11 and 17 years. However, the overall percentages at each age do mask some movement between categories – 7.6 % of children moved from overweight/obese to a normal BMI, and 7.0 % of students moved from normal weight to overweight/obese. A study of Belgian adolescents also supports the notion of limited increase in obesity prevalence after mid-childhood, which showed a stable prevalence between ages 13 and 17 years (Hulens et al. 2001).

Not all the evidence agrees about the stabilisation of obesity prevalence after mid-childhood. For example in an analysis of 2,379 school children in the USA, Kimm et al. showed that the prevalence of both overweight and obesity continued to rise from ages 9–19 years in both black and white females, with very large increases in the late teenage years (Kimm et al. 2002). At age nine 30.6 % of black females and 22.4 % of white females were overweight, rising to 39.3 % and 24.1 % respectively at age 16 and 56.9 % and 41.3 % at age 19.

A number of studies have also examined factors that affect the age of obesity onset, for example finding that maternal obesity (Gordon-Larsen et al. 2007), black ethnicity (Gordon-Larsen et al. 2007), and genetic factors (Hinney et al. 2007) are associated with younger age at becoming overweight/obese.

Thus overall, the evidence suggests rises in the mean level of age-adjusted adiposity and in the prevalence of overweight and obesity from birth across childhood until at least age 11, with some conflicting evidence over whether or not obesity prevalence stabilises after age 11 or rises further across adolescence. This suggests that there is no one age range of childhood and adolescence that should be the main focus of preventative interventions. However, in addition to considering the age distribution of obesity onset, decisions about the timing of interventions should also consider the likely success of intervening at different ages, cost-effectiveness of alternative policies, and the age at which health complications of obesity begin to develop. In relation to cardiovascular disease, childhood adiposity from around age 7–9 is what appears to matter, with weak, inverse or null associations at younger ages (Owen et al. 2009). It is also important to remember that regardless of how obesity prevalence changes across childhood and adolescence, some people will remain in the healthy BMI range across the whole of childhood but become overweight or obese as adults (Whitlock et al. 2005). For example, in a study in which 1,520 people were followed-up over ten years from the age of 14 (Patton et al. 2011), 33 % of participants were overweight (BMI $\geq$25 kg/m^2) at the end of the study (age 24 years). Of these, approximately 40 % had been consistently in the normal BMI range during adolescence, and approximately 80 % had at least one BMI measurement in the normal range at some point during the ten years of follow-up. Approximately half of the obese 24 year-olds had never been classified as obese during adolescence. Various life course events during adulthood have been shown to be associated with adiposity gains in adulthood, including pregnancy (Fraser et al.

2011), suggesting that these may be sensitive periods in adulthood and potentially suitable timings for preventative interventions (Tanentsapf et al. 2011).

Once a Child Becomes Overweight or Obese, How Likely is He/She to Remain So?

Understanding the incidence of overweight and obesity only tells part of the story – the degree of stability or persistence of overweight is also important, i.e. once a child becomes overweight or obese, how likely is he/she to remain so? This concept is referred to as 'tracking' in the epidemiological literature. Information on the degree of tracking of overweight and obesity is valuable for public health planning, since it informs the need for and likely long-term efficacy of preventative interventions in childhood.

A systematic review of the degree of tracking of overweight between childhood or adolescence into adulthood was published in 2008 (Singh et al.). The review included papers listed in MEDLINE, EMBASE and CINAHL up to February 2007. Publications were included if they reported at least one anthropometric measurement during youth (≤ 18 years) and one anthropometric measurement during adulthood (≥ 19 years), using body mass index (BMI), skin fold thickness or waist circumference to define body weight status in a general population study (i.e. excluding follow-up of intervention studies or studies in specific clinical populations or those concentrating only on a population that had experienced a certain exposure). Studies had to report an odds ratio (OR) or risk ratio (RR) for overweight youth becoming overweight adults. From the searches, the authors identified 18 studies described in 25 publications. All of these studies found that being overweight or obese during youth was associated with an increased risk of being overweight or obese in adulthood (Singh et al. 2008).

Four studies included in the systematic review stratified their analysis by weight status in childhood and all found that the odds of persistent overweight/obesity were greater with increasing level of overweight. When studies included more than one measure of overweight/obesity during youth, most found that the degree of tracking was greater at older ages – this could represent stronger tracking at older ages or may be a result of the shorter time intervals between the measurement in youth and measurement in adulthood, or of height changing less at older ages.

There was a considerable degree of heterogeneity in the estimates of the degree of tracking of overweight/obesity from youth into adulthood. The authors rates each included study as 'high' or 'low' methodological quality based on whether they met a list of pre-defined criteria for the conduct and reporting of observational studies. Amongst studies rated as high-quality, relative risks for overweight children becoming overweight adults ranged from 2 to 10. Relative risks for obese youth becoming obese adults were generally higher. Heterogeneity between studies may have arisen for multiple reasons: the studies were based in different populations with varying levels of obesity, ages of measurement in both youth and adulthood varied considerably, measurement protocols and definitions of overweight and obesity varied, as did statistical analysis procedures. The studies included in this systematic review are necessarily limited to populations who are now adults; it is therefore possible that the degree of tracking of overweight and obesity from childhood into adult may differ in younger populations who are growing up now, during the obesity epidemic, and in the future. A further consideration is that all studies included in the review were conducted in high-income countries, and so the extent of tracking within low- and middle-income countries is largely unknown.

In addition to the findings about persistence of overweight and obesity from childhood into adulthood described above, studies have also looked at tracking *within* childhood and adolescence. Amongst 2,747 female and 2,488 male participants of ALSPAC, the majority (70.7 % of females, 74.6 % of males) had a BMI within the normal range at both 9–12 and 15 years, whilst 13.4 % of females and 12.2 % of males were overweight/obese at both ages (Lawlor et al. 2010). Amongst female participants, 11.1 % moved from being overweight/obese at age 9–12 to normal BMI at age 15, and 4.8 % moved from normal BMI to overweight/obese; these percentages were 9.1 % and 4.1 % in males. Thus in this population, between 9–12 and 15 years, a greater number of children moved from being overweight/obese to having a normal BMI than developed obesity. Wright et al. carried out further analyses of ALSPAC data, looking at the tracking of body composition between ages seven and 11 using BMI and leg-to-leg bioelectrical impedance (BIA) (Wright et al. 2010). The BIA data were used to generate measures of lean and fat mass independent of height, gender and age, which were then internally standardised, with the 85th and 95th centiles considered as over-fat and very over-fat. In the more than 6,000 children included in their analysis, Wright et al. showed that of the children who were overweight by BMI at age seven, 21 % had reverted to a normal BMI by age 11 and 16 % had become obese. Using the BIA data, of those children who were over-fat at age seven, 12 % progressed to being very over-fat at age 11, 33 % remained over-fat and 55 % dropped to the normal fat category. Of the children who were very over-fat at age seven, 57 % remained so at age 11, 30 % dropped to over-fat and 13 % dropped to the normal fat category. There was therefore a slightly higher degree of tracking when using BMI as the measure of adiposity compared with BIA-assessed fat mass. In a separate analysis of ALSPAC data, Reilly et al. (2011) showed that 34 % of overweight (by BMI) children at age seven become obese by age 13. The OR for progression from overweight at age seven to obese at age 13 was 18.1 (95 % CI 12.8–25.6).

Wardle et al. followed more than 5,000 school children in London between the ages of 11 and 15 years (Wardle et al. 2006). The year to year correlations between BMI measurements were extremely high – 0.94 for a one year interval, reducing to 0.90, 0.86, and 0.82 for two, three, and four year intervals. A similar degree of tracking was observed for measurements of waist circumference, with correlations going from 0.86 for a one year interval between measurements to 0.70 for a four year interval. Using correlation coefficients to assess tracking can, however, be problematic since large correlations can arise even in the absence of strong tracking if the average slope over time is low.

Several studies have examined factors that may affect the degree of tracking of adiposity. There is little consistency in findings about whether or not tracking differs between males and females (Singh et al. 2008). Some evidence suggests a stronger degree of tracking in overweight children whose parents are obese (Wright et al. 2010). Socioeconomic position (SEP) and ethnicity, both known to be associated with childhood obesity (El-Sayed et al. 2011, 2012; Singh et al. 2010), may also affect tracking. One small Danish study (N = 384) found that low SEP participants were twice as likely to maintain overweight between ages 8–10 years and 14–16 years compared with high SEP participants, and twice as likely to develop overweight between the two time points (Kristensen et al. 2006). Analyses of the ALSPAC cohort found that there were no clear maternal education differences in the proportion of overweight seven year-olds becoming obese by age 15. There was, however, some indication that normal BMI seven year olds were slightly more likely to become overweight by age 15 if they were from lower maternal education categories, and children from higher maternal education categories are more likely to return from overweight/obese at age seven to a normal BMI at age 15 compared with children from lower maternal education groups (Howe 2013). A study looking at racial differences in overweight/obesity tracking between childhood and adulthood in a biracial cohort in the USA found that, despite initial BMI being similar in black and white children (aged 5–14 years), BMI increased more with age in black than white individuals, and overweight black children were more likely to become obese adults (84 % of black girls compared with 65 % of white girls, with similar findings in males) (Freedman et al. 2005).

In addition to tracking of adiposity itself, studies have also revealed persistence of obesity-related behaviours across childhood and adolescence. In a study of 296 children in Victoria, Australia, parents reported their child's television viewing and consumption of frequency of fruit, vegetable, and energy-dense sweet and savoury snacks in 2002/3 and again in 2006 and 2008 (Pearson et al. 2011). Standardised stability coefficients (interpreted as correlation coefficients, i.e. ranging from 0 (no relationship) to 1 (perfect relationship)) between the three time points ranged from 0.65 to 0.73 for television viewing, 0.52 to 0.86 for vegetable consumption, 0.73 to 0.89 for fruit consumption, 0.41 to 0.65 for consumption of energy-dense sweet snacks, and 0.40 to 0.67 for consumption of energy-dense savoury snacks. No consistent differences in tracking were seen between males and females or between children who were five to six or 10 to 12 at baseline.

Jones et al. (2013) conducted a systematic review of tracking of physical activity and sedentary behaviour within early childhood (between birth and age six years) or between early childhood and mid-childhood (6–12 years). Eleven studies were included in their review. The reported tracking coefficients for physical activity were moderate in the majority (60 %) of studies, with just 4 % of studies reporting high tracking; the considerable degree of measurement error in physical activity data may, however, contribute to the apparently moderate tracking. There was a greater degree of tracking for sedentary behaviour, with 33 % of studies reporting high tracking, and a further 50 % reporting moderate tracking. A further review demonstrated a moderate degree of tracking of sedentary behaviours within young people (Biddle et al. 2010). The authors identified 21 studies, with tracking coefficients from 0.08 to 0.73 for TV viewing, from 0.18 to 0.52 for electronic game/computer use, from 0.16 to 0.65 for total screen time, and from −0.15 to 0.48 for total sedentary time. Tracking coefficients tended to be higher with shorter intervals between measurements. Telema (2009) carried out a systematic review of the stability of physical activity from childhood into adulthood, reporting statistically significant evidence of tracking of physical activity levels across the life course, but with only a moderate degree of tracking between most periods of life and lower tracking in transition periods such as between adolescence and adulthood. The review also indicated that tracking tended to be lower in females compared with males.

Thus in conclusion, there is evidence for a moderate to strong degree of tracking across childhood and adolescence and between childhood and adulthood for both adiposity itself and adiposity-related behaviours such as diet, physical activity and sedentary behaviours. There is, however, some degree of movement both into and out of obesity at all stages of the life course, highlighting the need for preventative interventions across the life course.

Aetiological Insight from Studying Childhood Adiposity Trajectories

Longitudinal analyses of trajectories of adiposity across childhood and adolescence can be extremely useful for advancing our understanding of the aetiology of obesity and its long term health complications. One important scientific question that can only be addressed with life course studies is the extent to which one's obesity history matters for health – i.e. is final attained level of adiposity the key determinant of health, or do different life course adiposity patterns that converge on the same final size have varying health consequences? In the case of childhood obesity, a related question is the extent to which the long-term health sequelae of increased adiposity during childhood are due to permanent and irreversible damage to organs and tissues as a result of being overweight as a child, or the extent to which these associations are driven by tracking of adiposity levels such that overweight children tend to become overweight adults, with damage to tissues and organs only taking place in adulthood. These two scenarios have very different public health implications. In the first instance, if being overweight or obese as a child results in permanent damage to bodily systems, the public health impetus might be on preventing the development of obesity. However, if the second theory is correct and associations between childhood obesity and health in later life are driven solely by the tracking of adiposity, interventions that treat obesity in adulthood could potentially be as effective for preventing disease as those that prevent the development of obesity. Of course other factors need to be considered in this equation, including the cost and effectiveness of both types of intervention.

The evidence for these alternative hypotheses is somewhat mixed. There is now a very large body of evidence demonstrating that increased adiposity is cross-sectionally and prospectively associated with adverse cardiometabolic health even in very young children, using measures such as circulating levels of insulin, glucose or lipids, or even measurements of the structure and function of the heart (de Jonge et al. 2011; Falaschetti et al. 2010). However, two recent studies provide some encouraging evidence that obese children who normalise their weight status can also improve their cardiometabolic health. In analyses of 5,235 participants of the ALSPAC cohort, prospective associations were demonstrated between BMI, waist circumference and DXA-assessed total body fat mass at age 9–12 years and cardiovascular risk factors (systolic and diastolic blood pressure, concentrations of fasting glucose, insulin, triglycerides, low density lipoprotein cholesterol and high density lipoprotein cholesterol) assessed at age 15–16 years (Lawlor et al. 2010). Females in the cohort who were overweight or obese at ages 9–12 but whose BMI was in the normal range at ages 15–16 had similar odds of adverse levels of cardiometabolic risk factors to those females who were normal BMI at both ages. This pattern was less evident in males; males who normalised their BMI status between the two time points had higher odds of high systolic blood pressure, high concentrations of triglycerides and insulin, and low concentrations of high density lipoprotein cholesterol compared with those who were normal BMI at both ages, but their odds of having adverse levels of all cardiometabolic risk factors were lower than in those who remained overweight/obese at both ages. The continued elevated cardiometabolic risk in these males may be due to greater adiposity; mean BMI was higher in those who were overweight or obese at the first time point and had a BMI in the normal range at the second time point compared with those whose BMI was in the normal range at both ages. A similar research question was addressed in a study of 6,328 participants from four studies with a mean age of measurement in childhood of 11.4 years (SD = 4.0) and follow-up in adulthood on average 23.1 years later (SD = 3.3 years) (Juonala et al. 2011). The authors showed that participants who had been overweight or obese during childhood but whose BMI was in the normal range during adulthood have a similar risk of type 2 diabetes, hypertension, adverse levels of LDL-cholesterol, HDL-cholesterol, triglycerides, and an adverse carotid artery intima-media thickness as compared with participants whose BMI was in the normal range during both childhood and adulthood. Both of these studies therefore provide encouraging evidence that childhood obesity may not in itself cause permanent and irreversible damage to cardiometabolic systems, and that interventions that are successful in treating and reversing childhood obesity may be expected to improve the long-term cardiometabolic health of those people who are successfully treated.

The study by Juonala et al. (2011) also showed a similar level of cardiometabolic risk in participants who were overweight or obese in both childhood and adulthood as compared with participants who had a normal BMI during childhood but were overweight or obese as adults, suggesting that it may be the final attained adiposity level that influences cardiovascular health, and that the trajectory a person has followed to reach that level may be less important. Other studies, however, do not all support this hypothesis. For instance there is evidence that the duration of obesity is associated with mortality independent of BMI level. Abdullah et al. (2011) conducted analysis of 5,036 participants from the Framingham cohort study. Using data from 48 years of follow-up, they showed that the adjusted hazard ratio for mortality increased with the number of years of obesity; compared with those who were never obese, being obese for 1–4.9, 5–14.9, 15–24.9, and ≥25 years was associated with adjusted hazard ratios for all-cause mortality of 1.51 (95 % confidence interval (CI) 1.27–1.79), 1.94 (95 % CI 1.71–2.20), 2.25 (95 % CI 1.89–2.67) and 2.52 (95 % CI 2.08–3.06), respectively. Similar patterns were found for cause-specific mortality from cardiovascular disease and cancer. The relationships were robust to adjustment for current BMI, and were reduced but not completely eliminated by adjustment for potential intermediate factors such as incident cardiovascular disease and diabetes or biomedical risk factors.

A large body of research has focused on the topic of whether infancy is a sensitive period in the development of obesity and cardiovascular research. Several studies have concluded that rapid growth in infancy is importantly associated with subsequent obesity and adverse cardiovascular health (Ong et al. 2000, 2009; Ong and Loos 2006). However, these studies have generally only examined changes in weight (or weight adjusted for height) during infancy, and have not considered the associations of growth in later periods of childhood with the same outcomes. Without these comparisons (i.e. determining whether weight change in infancy is more strongly associated with later outcomes than is weight change in later childhood) it is difficult to conclude that infancy is a sensitive period. Studies on this topic have used a variety of statistical methods, often less than ideal (Tilling et al. 2011c; Tu et al. 2013) – for instance, relying on repeated z-scores, an approach which does not model the clustering of measurements within individuals and generally can only include people with complete, non-missing, data at all ages. In ALSPAC and Probit, two large studies with lots of repeated measurements of growth, we have used multilevel models to define growth trajectories across childhood (Howe et al. 2013c; Tilling et al. 2011b); an approach which is appropriate for repeated measures data and which can incorporate missing data under a missing at random assumption. In these analyses, we have not found strong support for infancy as a sensitive period in relation to a wide range of cardiometabolic risk factors, including blood pressure (central and peripheral), glucose, lipids, insulin, and non-alcoholic fatty liver disease (Howe et al. 2010; Tilling et al. 2011a; Anderson et al. 2014).

Longitudinal studies also permit in-depth examination of the ways in which the determinants of obesity act throughout the life course, potentially providing deeper aetiological insight than would be possible in cross-sectional studies. For example, genome-wide association studies have identified genetic variants that are associated with obesity and greater BMI in adulthood. Since BMI changes in childhood can result from changes in both height and weight, examining the effect of the genetic variants on growth trajectories in childhood can provide improved understanding of the potential mechanisms through which the genes are acting (Paternoster et al. 2011; Warrington et al. 2013; Cousminer et al. 2013). Risk scores of obesity-related genetic variants have been shown to be associated with changes in height, weight and BMI across infancy and childhood, with the magnitude of associations changing across the life course (Warrington et al. 2013; Elks et al. 2010, 2012; Hardy et al. 2010). Similar analyses have also been conducted for trajectories of height and blood pressure across childhood and adolescence (Howe et al. 2013a; Paternoster et al. 2011). Longitudinal studies have also provided insight into inter-generational and cross-cohort differences in patterns of growth (Li et al. 2008; Li et al. 2009), and the influence of social determinants on the development of obesity risk (Kakinami et al. 2014; Ding and Gebel 2012; Walsemann et al. 2012); for example analysis of the ALSPAC cohort demonstrated that maternal education differences in offspring BMI begin at an earlier age for females than for males and widen across childhood (Howe et al. 2011), and a study of the Born in Bradford cohort showed that despite lighter birth weights, Pakistani infants gain weight and length quicker than white infants, indicating that the greater risk of obesity in the British Pakistani population may have its origins in very early life (Fairley et al. 2013).

Concluding Remarks

In this chapter, we have shown that life course studies of childhood obesity can offer insight into whether the incidence of obesity differs between periods of childhood and adolescence, and the degree to which childhood overweight and obesity persists across the life course, and we have discussed the utility of such information in assessing the potential consequences of targeting obesity prevention interventions at specific age groups. Our review of the literature concluded that incidence of overweight and obesity was high across all ages, and that despite some movement between categories, children who become overweight or obese are likely to remain overweight or obese. Together, this body of evidence suggests that obesity prevention policies should target all ages. We have also shown that longitudinal studies can provide deeper understanding of aetiological questions than is possible in cross-sectional studies – for instance such studies can evaluate whether the life course adiposity trajectory influences health independently of the final attained adiposity level, or can provide insight into the timing and mechanisms through which determinants of obesity exert their influence. As with all life course studies, research on the life course epidemiology of childhood obesity faces methodological challenges (Davey Smith et al. 2009; Davey Smith et al. 2007; Ness et al. 2011; Howe et al. 2013b). Cohort effects are likely to be considerable – today's children are growing up in an environment that is far more obesogenic than the environment experienced by today's adults. Continued study of new cohorts is therefore crucial (Cooper et al. 2012), as is utilising innovative methodological tools such as Mendelian Randomization (Davey Smith et al. 2009; Lawlor et al. 2008; Palmer et al. 2012), cross-cohort comparisons (Brion et al. 2011) and family-based designs (Brion 2013; Howe et al. 2012; Lawlor and Mishra 2009) that improve the strength of causal inference that can be reached from observational data. Given the growing burden of non-communicable diseases in low- and middle-income settings (Miranda et al. 2008), life course studies in these settings are also important, since the vast majority of literature in this area to date comes from high-income countries, and the findings do not necessarily generalise.

References

Abdullah, A., Wolfe, R., Stoelwinder, J. U., De Courten, M., Stevenson, C., Walls, H. L., & Peeters, A. (2011). The number of years lived with obesity and the risk of all-cause and cause-specific mortality. *International Journal of Epidemiology, 40*, 985–996.

Anderson, E. L., Howe, L. D., Fraser, A., Callaway, M. P., Sattar, N., Day, C., Tilling, K., & Lawlor, D. A. (2014). Weight trajectories through infancy and childhood and risk of non-alcoholic fatty liver disease in adolescence: The ALSPAC study. *Journal of Hepatology, 61*(3), 626–632.

Ara, R., Blake, L., Gray, L., Hernandez, M., Crowther, M., Dunkley, A., Warren, F., Jackson, R., Rees, A., Stevenson, M., Abrams, K., Cooper, N., Davies, M., Khunti, K., & Sutton, A. (2012). What is the clinical effectiveness and cost-effectiveness of using drugs in treating obese patients in primary care? A systematic review. *Health Technology Assessment, 16*, iii–xiv. 1–195.

Biddle, S. J., Pearson, N., Ross, G. M., & Braithwaite, R. (2010). Tracking of sedentary behaviours of young people: A systematic review. *Preventive Medicine, 51*, 345–351.

Brion, M. J. (2013). Commentary: Can maternal-paternal comparisons contribute to our understanding of maternal pre-pregnancy obesity and its association with offspring cognitive outcomes? *International Journal of Epidemiology, 42*, 518–519.

Brion, M. J., Lawlor, D. A., Matijasevich, A., Horta, B., Anselmi, L., Araujo, C. L., Menezes, A. M., Victora, C. G., & Smith, G. D. (2011). What are the causal effects of breastfeeding on IQ, obesity and blood pressure? Evidence from comparing high-income with middle-income cohorts. *International Journal of Epidemiology, 40*, 670–680.

Cooper, C., Frank, J., Leyland, A., Hardy, R., Lawlor, D. A., Wareham, N. J., Dezateux, C., & Inskip, H. (2012). Using cohort studies in lifecourse epidemiology. *Public Health, 126*, 190–192.

Cousminer, D. L., Berry, D. J., Timpson, N. J., Ang, W., Thiering, E., Byrne, E. M., Taal, H. R., Huikari, V., Bradfield, J. P., Kerkhof, M., Groen-Blokhuis, M. M., Kreiner-Moller, E., Marinelli, M., Holst, C., Leinonen, J. T., Perry, J. R., Surakka, I., Pietilainen, O., Kettunen, J., Anttila, V., Kaakinen, M., Sovio, U., Pouta, A., Das, S., Lagou, V., Power, C., Prokopenko, I., Evans, D. M., Kemp, J. P., Stpourcain, B., Ring, S., Palotie, A., Kajantie, E., Osmond, C., Lehtimaki, T., Viikari, J. S., Kahonen, M., Warrington, N. M., Lye, S. J., Palmer, L. J., Tiesler, C. M., Flexeder, C., Montgomery, G. W., Medland, S. E., Hofman, A., Hakonarson, H., Guxens, M., Bartels, M., Salomaa, V., Murabito, J. M., Kaprio, J., Sorensen, T. I., Ballester, F., Bisgaard, H., Boomsma, D. I., Koppelman, G. H., Grant, S. F., Jaddoe, V. W., Martin, N. G., Heinrich, J., Pennell, C. E., Raitakari, O. T., Eriksson, J. G., Smith, G. D., Hypponen, E., Jarvelin, M. R., Mccarthy, M. I., Ripatti, S., & Widen, E. (2013). Genome-wide association and longitudinal analyses reveal genetic loci linking pubertal height growth, pubertal timing and childhood adiposity. *Human Molecular Genetics, 22*, 2735–2747.

Datar, A., Shier, V., & Sturm, R. (2011). Changes in body mass during elementary and middle school in a national cohort of kindergarteners. *Pediatrics, 128*, e1411–e1417.

Davey Smith, G., Lawlor, D. A., Harbord, R., Timpson, N., Day, I., & Ebrahim, S. (2007). Clustered environments and randomized genes: a fundamental distinction between conventional and genetic epidemiology. *PLoS Medicine, 4*, e352.

Davey Smith, G., Leary, S., Ness, A., & Lawlor, D. A. (2009). Challenges and novel approaches in the epidemiological study of early life influences on later disease. *Advances in Experimental Medicine and Biology, 646,* 1–14.

De Jonge, L. L., Van Osch-Gevers, L., Willemsen, S. P., Steegers, E. A., Hofman, A., Helbing, W. A., & Jaddoe, V. W. (2011). Growth, obesity, and cardiac structures in early childhood: The generation r study. *Hypertension, 57,* 934–940.

Dietz, W. H. (2004). Overweight in childhood and adolescence. *New England Journal of Medicine, 350,* 855–857.

Ding, D., & Gebel, K. (2012). Built environment, physical activity, and obesity: What have we learned from reviewing the literature? *Health & Place, 18,* 100–105.

Elks, C. E., Loos, R. J., Sharp, S. J., Langenberg, C., Ring, S. M., Timpson, N. J., Ness, A. R., Davey Smith, G., Dunger, D. B., Wareham, N. J., & Ong, K. K. (2010). Genetic markers of adult obesity risk are associated with greater early infancy weight gain and growth. *PLoS Medicine, 7,* e1000284.

Elks, C. E., Loos, R. J., Hardy, R., Wills, A. K., Wong, A., Wareham, N. J., Kuh, D., & Ong, K. K. (2012). Adult obesity susceptibility variants are associated with greater childhood weight gain and a faster tempo of growth: The 1946 British birth cohort study. *The American Journal of Clinical Nutrition, 95,* 1150–1156.

El-Sayed, A. M., Scarborough, P., & Galea, S. (2011). Ethnic inequalities in obesity among children and adults in the UK: A systematic review of the literature. *Obesity Reviews, 12,* e516–e534.

El-Sayed, A. M., Scarborough, P., & Galea, S. (2012). Socioeconomic inequalities in childhood obesity in the United Kingdom: A systematic review of the literature. *Obesity Facts, 5,* 671–692.

Fairley, L., Petherick, E. S., Howe, L. D., Tilling, K., Cameron, N., Lawlor, D. A., West, J., & Wright, J. (2013). Describing differences in weight and length growth trajectories between white and Pakistani infants in the UK: Analysis of the born in Bradford birth cohort study using multilevel linear spline models. *Archives of Disease in Childhood, 98,* 274–279.

Falaschetti, E., Hingorani, A. D., Jones, A., Charakida, M., Finer, N., Whincup, P., Lawlor, D. A., Davey Smith, G., Sattar, N., & Deanfield, J. E. (2010). Adiposity and cardiovascular risk factors in a large contemporary population of pre-pubertal children. *European Heart Journal, 31,* 3063–3072.

Flegal, K. M., & Troiano, R. P. (2000). Changes in the distribution of body mass index of adults and children in the US population. *International Journal of Obesity and Related Metabolic Disorders, 24,* 807–818.

Fraser, A., Tilling, K., Macdonald-Wallis, C., Hughes, R., Sattar, N., Nelson, S. M., & Lawlor, D. A. (2011). Associations of gestational weight gain with maternal body mass index, waist circumference, and blood pressure measured 16 y after pregnancy: The Avon Longitudinal Study of Parents and Children (ALSPAC). *The American Journal of Clinical Nutrition, 93,* 1285–1292.

Freedman, D. S., Khan, L. K., Serdula, M. K., Dietz, W. H., Srinivasan, S. R., & Berenson, G. S. (2005). Racial differences in the tracking of childhood BMI to adulthood. *Obesity Research, 13,* 928–935.

Friedemann, C., Heneghan, C., Mahtani, K., Thompson, M., Perera, R., & Ward, A. M. (2012). Cardiovascular disease risk in healthy children and its association with body mass index: Systematic review and meta-analysis. *BMJ, 345,* e4759.

Gardner, D. S., Hosking, J., Metcalf, B. S., Jeffery, A. N., Voss, L. D., & Wilkin, T. J. (2009). Contribution of early weight gain to childhood overweight and metabolic health: A longitudinal study (EarlyBird 36). *Pediatrics, 123,* e67–e73.

Gordon-Larsen, P., Adair, L. S., & Suchindran, C. M. (2007). Maternal obesity is associated with younger age at obesity onset in U.S. Adolescent offspring followed into adulthood. *Obesity (Silver Spring), 15,* 2790–2796.

Han, J. C., Lawlor, D. A., & Kimm, S. Y. S. (2010). Childhood obesity. *Lancet, 375,* 1737–1748.

Hannon, T. S., Rao, G., & Arslanian, S. A. (2005). Childhood obesity and type 2 diabetes mellitus. *Pediatrics, 116*, 473–480.

Hardy, R., Wills, A. K., Wong, A., Elks, C. E., Wareham, N. J., Loos, R. J., Kuh, D., & Ong, K. K. (2010). Life course variations in the associations between FTO and MC4R gene variants and body size. *Human Molecular Genetics, 19*, 545–552.

Hinney, A., Nguyen, T. T., Scherag, A., Friedel, S., Bronner, G., Muller, T. D., Grallert, H., Illig, T., Wichmann, H. E., Rief, W., Schafer, H., & Hebebrand, J. (2007). Genome wide association (GWA) study for early onset extreme obesity supports the role of fat mass and obesity associated gene (FTO) variants. *PLoS ONE, 2*, e1361.

Howe, L. D. (2013). Childhood obesity: Socioeconomic inequalities and consequences for later cardiovascular health. *Longitudinal and Life Course Studies, 4*, 4–16.

Howe, L. D., Tilling, K., Benfield, L., Logue, J., Sattar, N., Ness, A. R., Smith, G. D., & Lawlor, D. A. (2010). Changes in ponderal index and body mass index across childhood and their associations with fat mass and cardiovascular risk factors at age 15. *PLoS ONE, 5*, e15186.

Howe, L. D., Tilling, K., Galobardes, B., Smith, G. D., Ness, A. R., & Lawlor, D. A. (2011). Socioeconomic disparities in trajectories of adiposity across childhood. *International Journal of Pediatric Obesity, 6*, e144–e153.

Howe, L. D., Matijasevich, A., Tilling, K., Brion, M. J., Leary, S. D., Smith, G. D., & Lawlor, D. A. (2012). Maternal smoking during pregnancy and offspring trajectories of height and adiposity: Comparing maternal and paternal associations. *International Journal of Epidemiology, 41*, 722–732.

Howe, L. D., Parmar, P. G., Paternoster, L., Warrington, N. M., Kemp, J. P., Briollais, L., Newnham, J. P., Timpson, N. J., Smith, G. D., Ring, S. M., Evans, D. M., Tilling, K., Pennell, C. E., Beilin, L. J., Palmer, L. J., & Lawlor, D. A. (2013a). Genetic influences on trajectories of systolic blood pressure across childhood and adolescence. *Circulation. Cardiovascular Genetics, 6*, 608–614.

Howe, L. D., Tilling, K., Galobardes, B., & Lawlor, D. A. (2013b). Loss to follow-up in cohort studies: Bias in estimates of socioeconomic inequalities. *Epidemiology, 24*, 1–9.

Howe, L. D., Tilling, K., Matijasevich, A., Petherick, E. S., Santos, A. C., Fairley, L., Wright, J., Santos, I. S., Barros, A. J., Martin, R. M., Kramer, M. S., Bogdanovich, N., Matush, L., Barros, H., & Lawlor, D. A. (2013c) Linear spline multilevel models for summarising childhood growth trajectories: A guide to their application using examples from five birth cohorts. *Stat Methods Med Res.* doi:10.1177/0962280213503925. [Epub ahead of print]

Hughes, A. R., Sherriff, A., Lawlor, D. A., Ness, A. R., & Reilly, J. J. (2011a). Incidence of obesity during childhood and adolescence in a large contemporary cohort. *Preventive Medicine, 52*, 300–304.

Hughes, A. R., Sherriff, A., Lawlor, D. A., Ness, A. R., & Reilly, J. J. (2011b). Timing of excess weight gain in the Avon Longitudinal Study of Parents and Children (ALSPAC). *Pediatrics, 127*, e730–e736.

Hulens, M., Beunen, G., Claessens, A. L., Lefevre, J., Thomis, M., Philippaerts, R., Borms, J., Vrijens, J., Lysens, R., & Vansant, G. (2001). Trends in BMI among Belgian children, adolescents and adults from 1969 to 1996. *International Journal of Obesity and Related Metabolic Disorders, 25*, 395–399.

Jones, R. A., Hinkley, T., Okely, A. D., & Salmon, J. (2013). Tracking physical activity and sedentary behavior in childhood: A systematic review. *American Journal of Preventive Medicine, 44*, 651–658.

Juonala, M., Magnussen, C. G., Berenson, G. S., Venn, A., Burns, T. L., Sabin, M. A., Srinivasan, S. R., Daniels, S. R., Davis, P. H., Chen, W., Sun, C., Cheung, M., Viikari, J. S., Dwyer, T., & Raitakari, O. T. (2011). Childhood adiposity, adult adiposity, and cardiovascular risk factors. *The New England Journal of Medicine, 365*, 1876–1885.

Kakinami, L., Seguin, L., Lambert, M., Gauvin, L., Nikiema, B., & Paradis, G. (2014). Poverty's latent effect on adiposity during childhood: Evidence from a Quebec birth cohort. *Journal of Epidemiology & Community Health, 68*, 239–245.

Kimm, S. Y., Barton, B. A., Obarzanek, E., Mcmahon, R. P., Kronsberg, S. S., Waclawiw, M. A., Morrison, J. A., Schreiber, G. B., Sabry, Z. I., & Daniels, S. R. (2002). Obesity development during adolescence in a biracial cohort: The NHLBI growth and health study. *Pediatrics, 110,* e54.

Kipping, R. R., Jago, R., & Lawlor, D. A. (2008). Obesity in children. Part 1: Epidemiology, measurement, risk factors, and screening. *BMJ, 337,* a1824.

Kristensen, P. L., Wedderkopp, N., Moller, N. C., Andersen, L. B., Bai, C. N., & Froberg, K. (2006). Tracking and prevalence of cardiovascular disease risk factors across socio-economic classes: A longitudinal substudy of the European youth heart study. *BMC Public Health, 6,* 20.

Lawlor, D. A., & Mishra, G. D. (Eds.). (2009). *Family matters: Designing, analysing and understanding family-based studies in life-course epidemiology.* New York: Oxford University Press.

Lawlor, D. A., Harbord, R. M., Sterne, J. A., Timpson, N., & Davey Smith, G. (2008). Mendelian randomization: Using genes as instruments for making causal inferences in epidemiology. *Statistics in Medicine, 27,* 1133–1163.

Lawlor, D. A., Benfield, L., Logue, J., Tilling, K., Howe, L. D., Fraser, A., Cherry, L., Watt, P., Ness, A. R., Davey Smith, G., & Sattar, N. (2010). Association between general and central adiposity in childhood, and change in these, with cardiovascular risk factors in adolescence: Prospective cohort study. *BMJ, 341,* c6224.

Li, L., Hardy, R., Kuh, D., Lo Conte, R., & Power, C. (2008). Child-to-adult body mass index and height trajectories: A comparison of 2 British birth cohorts. *American Journal of Epidemiology, 168,* 1008–1015.

Li, L., Law, C., Lo Conte, R., & Power, C. (2009). Intergenerational influences on childhood body mass index: The effect of parental body mass index trajectories. *The American Journal of Clinical Nutrition, 89,* 551–557.

Livhits, M., Mercado, C., Yermilov, I., Parikh, J. A., Dutson, E., Mehran, A., Ko, C. Y., & Gibbons, M. M. (2012). Preoperative predictors of weight loss following bariatric surgery: Systematic review. *Obesity Surgery, 22,* 70–89.

Loveman, E., Frampton, G. K., Shepherd, J., Picot, J., Cooper, K., Bryant, J., Welch, K., & Clegg, A. (2011). The clinical effectiveness and cost-effectiveness of long-term weight management schemes for adults: A systematic review. *Health Technology Assessment, 15,* 1–182.

Miranda, J. J., Kinra, S., Casas, J. P., Davey Smith, G., & Ebrahim, S. (2008). Non-communicable diseases in low- and middle-income countries: Context, determinants and health policy. *Tropical Medicine and International Health, 13,* 1225–1234.

Ness, A. R., Griffiths, A. E., Howe, L. D., & Leary, S. D. (2011). Drawing causal inferences in epidemiologic studies of early life influences. *The American Journal of Clinical Nutrition, 94,* 1959S–1963S.

Ogden, C. L., Carroll, M. D., Curtin, L. R., Lamb, M. M., & Flegal, K. M. (2010). Prevalence of high body mass index in US children and adolescents 2007–2008. *JAMA, 303,* 242–249.

Ong, K. K., & Loos, R. J. (2006). Rapid infancy weight gain and subsequent obesity: Systematic reviews and hopeful suggestions. *Acta Paediatrica, 95,* 904–908.

Ong, K. K., Ahmed, M. L., Emmett, P. M., Preece, M. A., & Dunger, D. B. (2000). Association between postnatal catch-up growth and obesity in childhood: Prospective cohort study. *BMJ, 320,* 967–971.

Ong, K. K., Emmett, P., Northstone, K., Golding, J., Rogers, I., Ness, A. R., Wells, J. C., & Dunger, D. B. (2009). Infancy weight gain predicts childhood body fat and age at menarche in girls. *Journal of Clinical Endocrinology and Metabolism, 94,* 1527–1532.

Owen, C. G., Whincup, P. H., Orfei, L., Chou, Q.-A., Rudnicka, A. R., Wathern, A. K., Kaye, S. J., Eriksson, J. G., Osmond, C., & Cook, D. G. (2009). Is body mass index before middle age related to coronary heart disease risk in later life? Evidence from observational studies. *International Journal of Obesity, 33,* 866–877.

Palmer, T. M., Lawlor, D. A., Harbord, R. M., Sheehan, N. A., Tobias, J. H., Timpson, N. J., Davey Smith, G., & Sterne, J. A. (2012). Using multiple genetic variants as instrumental variables for modifiable risk factors. *Statistical Methods in Medical Research, 21,* 223–242.

Parsons, T. J., Power, C., Logan, S., & Summerbell, C. D. (1999). Childhood predictors of adult obesity: A systematic review. *International Journal of Obesity and Related Metabolic Disorders, 23*(Supp 8), S1–S107.

Paternoster, L., Howe, L. D., Tilling, K., Weedon, M. N., Freathy, R. M., Frayling, T. M., Kemp, J. P., Smith, G. D., Timpson, N. J., Ring, S. M., Evans, D. M., & Lawlor, D. A. (2011). Adult height variants affect birth length and growth rate in children. *Human Molecular Genetics, 20*, 4069–4075.

Patton, G. C., Coffey, C., Carlin, J. B., Sawyer, S. M., Williams, J., Olsson, C. A., & Wake, M. (2011). Overweight and obesity between adolescence and young adulthood: A 10-year prospective cohort study. *The Journal of Adolescent Health, 48*, 275–280.

Pearson, N., Salmon, J., Campbell, K., Crawford, D., & Timperio, A. (2011). Tracking of children's body-mass index, television viewing and dietary intake over five-years. *Preventive Medicine, 53*, 268–270.

Picot, J., Jones, J., Colquitt, J. L., Gospodarevskaya, E., Loveman, E., Baxter, L., & Clegg, A. J. (2009). The clinical effectiveness and cost-effectiveness of bariatric (weight loss) surgery for obesity: A systematic review and economic evaluation. *Health Technology Assessment, 13*, 1–190. 215–357, iii-iv.

Public Health England. (2014) [Online]: http://www.noo.org.uk/NOO_about_obesity/obesity_ and_health. Accessed 13 Mar 2014.

Reilly, J. J., & Wilson, D. (2006). ABC of obesity. Childhood obesity. *BMJ, 333*, 1207–1210.

Reilly, J. J., Bonataki, M., Leary, S. D., Wells, J. C., Davey-Smith, G., Emmett, P., Steer, C., Ness, A. R., & Sherriff, A. (2011). Progression from childhood overweight to adolescent obesity in a large contemporary cohort. *International Journal of Pediatric Obesity, 6*, e138–e143.

Russell-Mayhew, S., Mcvey, G., Bardick, A., & Ireland, A. (2012). Mental health, wellness, and childhood overweight/obesity. *Journal of Obesity, 2012*, 281801.

Singh, A. S., Mulder, C., Twisk, J. W., Van Mechelen, W., & Chinapaw, M. J. (2008). Tracking of childhood overweight into adulthood: A systematic review of the literature. *Obesity Reviews, 9*, 474–488.

Singh, G. K., Siahpush, M., & Kogan, M. D. (2010). Rising social inequalities in US childhood obesity 2003–2007. *Annals of Epidemiology, 20*, 40–52.

Tanentsapf, I., Heitmann, B. L., & Adegboye, A. R. (2011). Systematic review of clinical trials on dietary interventions to prevent excessive weight gain during pregnancy among normal weight, overweight and obese women. *BMC Pregnancy and Childbirth, 11*, 81.

Telama, R. (2009). Tracking of physical activity from childhood to adulthood: A review. *Obesity Facts, 2*, 187–195.

Tilling, K., Davies, N., Windmeijer, F., Kramer, M. S., Bogdanovich, N., Matush, L., Patel, R., Smith, G. D., Ben-Shlomo, Y., & Martin, R. M. (2011a). Is infant weight associated with childhood blood pressure? Analysis of the Promotion of Breastfeeding Intervention Trial (PROBIT) cohort. *International Journal of Epidemiology, 40*, 1227–1237.

Tilling, K., Davies, N. M., Nicoli, E., Ben-Shlomo, Y., Kramer, M. S., Patel, R., Oken, E., & Martin, R. M. (2011b). Associations of growth trajectories in infancy and early childhood with later childhood outcomes. *The American Journal of Clinical Nutrition, 94*, 1808S–1813S.

Tilling, K., Howe, L. D., & Ben-Shlomo, Y. (2011c). Commentary: Methods for analysing life course influences on health–untangling complex exposures. *International Journal of Epidemiology, 40*, 250–252.

Tu, Y. K., Tilling, K., Sterne, J. A., & Gilthorpe, M. S. (2013). A critical evaluation of statistical approaches to examining the role of growth trajectories in the developmental origins of health and disease. *International Journal of Epidemiology, 42*, 1327–1339.

Von Hinke Kessler Scholder, S., Davey Smith, G., Lawlor, D. A., Propper, C., & Windmeijer, F. (2012). The effect of fat mass on educational attainment: Examining the sensitivity to different identification strategies. *Economics and Human Biology, 10*, 405–418.

Walsemann, K. M., Ailshire, J. A., Bell, B. A., & Frongillo, E. A. (2012). Body mass index trajectories from adolescence to midlife: Differential effects of parental and respondent education by race/ethnicity and gender. *Ethnicity and Health, 17*, 337–362.

Wang, Y., & Lobstein, T. (2006). Worldwide trends in childhood overweight and obesity. *International Journal of Pediatric Obesity, 1*, 11–25.

Wardle, J., Brodersen, N. H., Cole, T. J., Jarvis, M. J., & Boniface, D. R. (2006). Development of adiposity in adolescence: Five year longitudinal study of an ethnically and socioeconomically diverse sample of young people in Britain. *BMJ, 332*, 1130–1135.

Warrington, N. M., Howe, L. D., Wu, Y. Y., Timpson, N. J., Tilling, K., Pennell, C. E., Newnham, J., Davey-Smith, G., Palmer, L. J., Beilin, L. J., Lye, S. J., Lawlor, D. A., & Briollais, L. (2013). Association of a body mass index genetic risk score with growth throughout childhood and adolescence. *PLoS ONE, 8*, e79547.

Whitlock, E. P., Williams, S. B., Gold, R., Smith, P. R., & Shipman, S. A. (2005). Screening and interventions for childhood overweight: A summary of evidence for the US Preventive Services Task Force. *Pediatrics, 116*, e125–e144.

Wright, C. M., Emmett, P. M., Ness, A. R., Reilly, J. J., & Sherriff, A. (2010). Tracking of obesity and body fatness through mid-childhood. *Archives of Disease in Childhood, 95*, 612–617.

Chapter 3
Oral Health Over the Life Course

Anja Heilmann, Georgios Tsakos, and Richard G. Watt

Introduction

Oral health is an integral and core component of overall health and well-being. The main oral diseases include dental caries (tooth decay), periodontal disease (gum disease) and oral cancers, all of which are common chronic conditions that affect a considerable proportion of both the child and adult populations across the world. Oral diseases have been somewhat neglected by policy makers and politicians, and considered as a marginal health issue. However, at a recent United Nations summit on the prevention of non-communicable diseases, oral conditions were highlighted as a major global public health priority (UN 2011).

Dental caries and periodontal diseases are both highly prevalent chronic conditions. Caries can affect individuals across the life course from early childhood to old age. It is often stated that caries is the most common chronic disease in childhood. In the US, it is estimated that caries is five times as common as asthma and seven times as common as allergic rhinitis (Benjamin 2010). Caries is a cumulative condition, and prevalence increases with age. The recent Global Burden of Disease (GBD) 2010 Study found that untreated caries of the permanent dentition was the most prevalent condition worldwide, affecting 35 % of the global population (Marcenes et al. 2013). Periodontal disease largely affects adults and older people. Although most adults have some gingival inflammation (bleeding gums), approximately 11 % of the global adult population have severe progressive periodontal disease, which can ultimately lead to premature tooth loss (Marcenes et al. 2013). Rates of oral cancer, a debilitating and potentially fatal condition, are steadily increasing across

A. Heilmann (✉) • G. Tsakos • R.G. Watt
Department of Epidemiology and Public Health, University College London, London, UK
e-mail: anja.heilmann@ucl.ac.uk; g.tsakos@ucl.ac.uk; r.watt@ucl.ac.uk

© The Author(s) 2015
C. Burton-Jeangros et al. (eds.), *A Life Course Perspective on Health Trajectories and Transitions*, Life Course Research and Social Policies 4,
DOI 10.1007/978-3-319-20484-0_3

Europe. In the UK, 6,500 people are diagnosed each year with oral cancer, which is similar to the number of women affected by cervical cancer (Cancer Research UK 2012).

Despite being very common, oral diseases are largely preventable. However, oral diseases are socially patterned, with disadvantaged and lower income groups disproportionally affected (Hobdell et al. 2003). Indeed, consistent stepwise social gradients exist for both clinical and subjective oral health outcomes, at all points across the life course (Sheiham et al. 2011).

As well as being very common, oral diseases have a significant negative impact on quality of life and well being (Fig. 3.1). The recent global burden of disease study highlighted that oral diseases accounted for 15 million disability adjusted life years globally (Marcenes et al. 2013). In preschool children, caries in the primary dentition (baby teeth) is often left untreated, causing severe pain, discomfort and

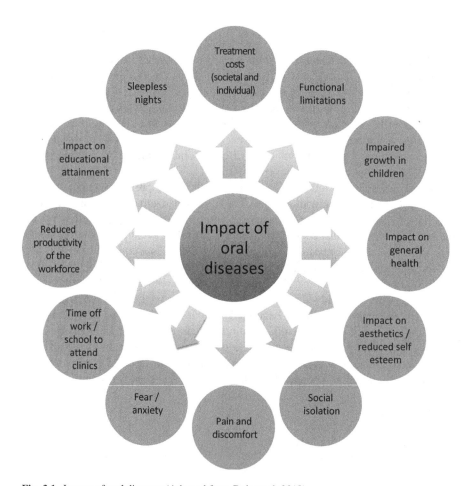

Fig. 3.1 Impact of oral diseases (Adapted from Daly et al. 2013)

infection (both acute and chronic). The resulting eating and sleep disruption can adversely affect children's ability to concentrate in school, ultimately compromising their educational performance (Sheiham 2006). Moreover, severe dental caries has been shown to negatively impact on a child's growth and development (Duijster et al. 2013; Sheiham 2006). Amongst adults and older people, tooth loss caused by dental caries or periodontal disease can severely restrict dietary intakes, particularly of fresh fruits and vegetables (Tsakos et al. 2010). Further, there is evidence for direct links between oral health and general health. Systematic reviews concluded that poor oral hygiene and periodontal disease are risk factors for pneumonia, and possibly also for chronic obstructive pulmonary disease (Azarpazhooh and Leake 2006; Sjögren et al. 2008), and that periodontal disease adversely affects diabetes outcomes (Borgnakke et al. 2013).

The treatment of caries is costly and time consuming. In the UK, the multiple extraction of carious teeth is the main reason for administering general anesthesia among young children, a costly and traumatic experience. In addition to the negative effect on the individual and their family, oral diseases also impose a major economic burden in terms of the costs to the health care system of providing dental treatment. WHO (2003) has estimated that dental care accounts for between 5 and 10 % of total healthcare expenditure and that dental caries is the fourth most expensive disease to treat. In addition to the direct costs of dental treatment, indirect costs are also very high. In the US, it is estimated that 2.4 million days of work were lost due to attendance at dental services for the treatment of oral diseases (Beaglehole et al. 2009).

From a clinical perspective, oral diseases are caused by poor oral hygiene, diets high in added sugars, lack of fluoride, tobacco use and excess alcohol consumption. It is increasingly recognised that oral diseases share common behavioural risks with the other main non-communicable conditions (Sheiham and Watt 2000; Watt and Sheiham 2012). For example, high sugars consumption is the main cause of dental caries, but is also linked with overweight and obesity (WHO 2003). However from a public health perspective, it is fundamentally important to acknowledge that behaviours are socially patterned and therefore shared health behaviours are enmeshed and determined by their broader social, environmental and political context. Health related behaviours alone do not account for patterns of oral diseases in the population. A broader social determinants framework which includes biological, behavioural, psychosocial, economic, environmental and political factors is now recognised as an appropriate approach to explore the aetiology of chronic diseases, including oral conditions and patterns of health inequalities (Marmot and Bell 2011).

As will be outlined in this chapter, oral diseases are ideal for the application of life course epidemiological research (Nicolau et al. 2007b). They are cumulative and chronic in nature, relatively common across the population and can be measured with good accuracy. In addition, they share common social determinants with other chronic non-communicable conditions, and indeed are a suitable early marker for exposure to risk factors across the life course.

Oral Health Over the Life Course: Evidence from Empirical Studies

Over the past decade, the number of published oral health studies adopting a life course perspective has been steadily increasing. Main lines of enquiry relate to critical period and accumulation of risk models, and include outcome measures such as developmental defects of enamel, levels of caries and periodontal disease, tooth loss and oral health-related quality of life (OHRQoL). Some studies have examined the interrelationships between oral and general health, such as the associations between caries experience and child growth. The following sections provide an overview of the most important findings on oral health over the life course so far.

Developmental Defects of Enamel

Dental enamel is the hardest tissue of the body. Its formation (amelogenesis) takes place over a time window starting prenatally and spanning the first years of life up to age 11, with specific timings depending on tooth type (Reid and Dean 2006). Enamel is formed incrementally and cyclically during tooth development. Similar to the rings of a tree, the periodical activity of enamel-secreting cells results in fine lines, the so-called Striae of Retzius, which can be seen on the enamel surface as grooves called perikymata (Figs. 3.2 and 3.3). In accordance with a critical

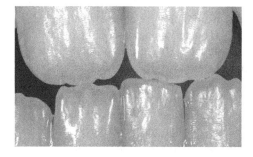

Fig. 3.2 Visible perikymata on the surface of dental enamel (Image courtesy of Dr Ali Golkari, Shiraz University of Medical Sciences, Iran)

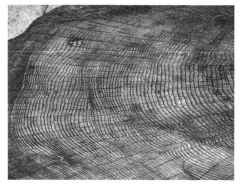

Fig. 3.3 Rings of a tree (Note: This is a Wikimedia image released unconditionally into the public domain, no copyright: http://en.wikipedia.org/wiki/File:Tree.ring.arp.jpg)

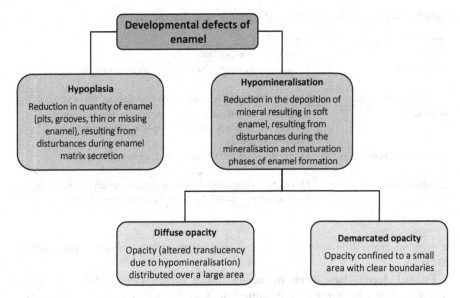

Fig. 3.4 Types of developmental defects of enamel (Adapted from Seow 2013)

period model, disturbances occurring during the development of dental enamel may result in visible and immutable defects. The microstructure of enamel therefore provides a fascinating record not only of the timing of tooth development, but also of any disturbances due to early life experiences. These features of enamel are used also in anthropological and evolutionary research (Dean 2006; Humphrey et al. 2008). Dental hard tissues can also provide important information on exposure to environmental pollution. For example, recent advances make it possible to assess lead levels accumulated over the first few years of life from exfoliated primary teeth.

The aetiology and implications of developmental defects of enamel (DDE) have been reviewed by Seow (2013). An overview of the classification of enamel defects is shown in Fig. 3.4. Enamel defects due to disturbances during the secretion phase result in enamel hypoplasia, a reduction in the quantity of enamel. Insults during the mineralisation and maturation phases manifest as enamel hypomineralisation, which becomes visible in the form of diffuse or demarcated opacities.

Enamel defects are caused by a range of factors including genetic conditions (Table 3.1). Of interest from a life course perspective are especially those influences that are acquired rather than hereditary. These include early malnutrition, metabolic disturbances, infections, exposure to chemicals or drugs and trauma, or combinations of these. Systemic factors will affect several teeth at the same time, depending on their developmental stage, while defects involving only single teeth point towards localised trauma such as from orotracheal intubation in preterm children. It is possible to deduce the timing of the insult from the type of defect, i.e. hypoplasia

Table 3.1 Main causes for developmental defects of enamel (Seow 2013)

Main causes	Examples
Genetic	Amelogenesis imperfecta
Malnutrition	Protein-energy malnutrition (PEM), Vitamin D deficiency (rickets)
Metabolic disturbances	Chronic renal and liver disease, coeliac disease, hypocalcaemia
Infections	Respiratory infections, chickenpox, rubella, measles, mumps, influenza, cytomegalovirus, meningococcal infection, congenital syphilis
Exposure to chemicals or drugs	Dental fluorosis, tetracyclines, lead, cytotoxic drugs
Localised trauma	Orotracheal intubation in preterm children, trauma to deciduous tooth affecting enamel development of permanent tooth

or hypomineralisation, and from its location on the tooth surface (Seow 1997, 2013).

Enamel defects have been frequently linked to low birth weight, an association that has been recently examined in a systematic review of 23 studies. The review concluded that there is currently good evidence for a relationship between very low birth weight and enamel opacities, and between preterm birth and enamel hypoplasia in primary teeth (baby teeth), while for permanent teeth the evidence was deemed inconclusive (Jacobsen et al. 2014). The main pathway is probably via mineral deficiencies resulting from the systemic conditions that are associated with low birth weight, such as malnutrition, gastrointestinal and renal disorders and severe infections (Seow 2013). Maternal risk factors related to low birth weight, such as smoking, have also been implicated in the aetiology of enamel defects (Needleman et al. 1992). Given that the risk of low birth weight is associated with socio-economic disadvantage (Kramer et al. 2000), it would be expected that the prevalence of enamel defects is socially graded. However, the question of a social gradient in relation to developmental defects of enamel has not been conclusively addressed in the literature.

The most important consequence of enamel defects is an increased susceptibility to dental caries, but aesthetic concerns and tooth sensitivity can also be considerable, and clinical management especially of children can be difficult and costly (Seow 2013). Thus, developmental defects of enamel may be viewed as one link in a chain of risk model, where early life stressors lead to enamel defects, which in turn are associated with a higher risk of dental caries. For the primary dentition, the particular pathway between early malnutrition and dental caries has been reviewed and generally supported, however high quality evidence from longitudinal studies is still needed (Psoter et al. 2005).

Early Life Conditions and Adult Oral Health

Most of the oral health research that explicitly made reference to a life course approach has examined childhood socio-economic characteristics in relation to adolescent or adult oral health. The paucity of prospective cohort studies that contain clinical data on oral health means that much of the longitudinal evidence currently available stems from only three birth cohort studies: the Newcastle Thousand Families 1947 birth cohort in England, the Dunedin Multidisciplinary Health and Development Study in New Zealand, whose members were born in 1972–1973, and the 1982 and 1993 Pelotas birth cohorts in Brazil. An alternative approach taken by a number of studies is the use of information collected retrospectively.

Childhood Socio-economic Background and Adult Levels of Disease

Three studies have analysed data from the Newcastle Thousand Families cohort to assess the relationships between childhood socio-economic status (SES) and tooth retention, as well as oral health-related quality of life, at 50 years of age (Mason et al. 2006; Pearce et al. 2004, 2009). Pearce et al. (2004) examined a sample of 337 participants to establish the relative importance of risk factors operating in childhood and adulthood for tooth retention at age 50. In this study, most of the variance in the number of retained teeth was explained by adult factors, namely socio-economic status, smoking and alcohol consumption. Childhood SES was predictive of tooth retention in middle age only among women, and this relationship was no longer statistically significant after adjustment for adult SES. In contrast, in the same sample oral health-related quality of life was associated with childhood SES only among men, and again the relationship was fully mediated by adult SES (Mason et al. 2006). For both men and women, the number of retained teeth to middle age was related to oral health-related quality of life.

These findings are in contrast to research that investigated the associations between childhood SES and levels of caries and periodontal disease at age 26 in the aforementioned Dunedin Study from New Zealand (Poulton et al. 2002; Thomson et al. 2004). Both studies in this younger cohort found that childhood SES contributed to adult levels of disease, after adjusting for adult SES. A study based on the Survey of Health, Ageing, and Retirement in Europe (SHARE), which used data from 13 European countries, reported that childhood financial hardship was an independent predictor of functional limitation (reduced chewing ability) at age 50 (Listl et al. 2014). Further, Nicolau et al. (2007a) reported an independent association between low paternal education in childhood and periodontal disease in adulthood among a small sample of women in Brazil.

The role of parental education as a measure of childhood socio-economic background was examined also in a study by Bernabé et al. (2011), who analysed data from 7,112 adult participants in the Finnish Health 2000 Survey. This study explicitly tested critical period and accumulation of risk models in relation to oral health. Outcome measures were edentulousness (total tooth loss), perceived oral health, dental caries and periodontal disease, measured in adulthood (the mean age of the sample was 53 years). Parental education was measured retrospectively, and models adjusted for participants' own level of education attained. The results supported all three life course models: both parental and own education contributed independently to adult oral health, with the exception of periodontal disease which was associated with own education only. Further, the study found a graded relationship between the level of cumulative exposure to low education and the four markers of oral health, in that oral health was poorest among those who were exposed to socio-economic disadvantage in both childhood and adulthood, followed by those who were exposed to disadvantage at only one time point, while those who were never in the low education group had the most favourable outcomes.

In the Dunedin Study, researchers also found evidence for intergenerational effects: adult caries experience at age 32 was related to maternal oral health measured at age 5 (Shearer et al. 2011). The relationship was graded across the categories of maternal self-rated oral health, with the highest caries risk found among those whose mothers had rated their oral health as poor or were edentulous, after adjusting for childhood SES and plaque trajectories. These findings are supported by results from a large cross-sectional study among more than 6,000 mother and child pairs in Quebec, Canada (Bedos et al. 2005). The Canadian data showed that caries experience among 5–9 year old children was associated with maternal edentulousness, independent of family socio-economic status, age, gender and children's oral health related behaviours such as toothbrushing, eating sugary snacks and dental visits. It is however likely that the behavioural variables adjusted for were too crude to fully explain the behavioural pathway, especially in relation to the role of dietary sugars. Similarly, parental dental status at age 10 was related to adult oral health among three different birth cohorts (born 1929–1938, 1939–1948 and 1959–1960) in Norway (Holst and Schuller 2012). To further corroborate intergenerational effects, a small study from the US among a low-income Hispanic cohort found that mothers' levels of cariogenic bacteria in their saliva were related to levels of caries experienced by their children (Chaffee et al. 2014). The authors suggest that the association is likely to be due to shared environmental factors, as well as direct maternal-to-child transfer of bacteria.

Impact of Social Mobility on Oral Health Outcomes

From accumulation of risk models it follows that health outcomes should be influenced by a reduction or increase in risk via upward or downward social mobility. Such social trajectories models have been investigated also in relation to oral health, however the findings so far have been somewhat mixed.

A study on the Newcastle Thousand Families cohort used information on social class at age 25, retrospectively collected at age 50, to test associations between markers of oral health and upward and downward social mobility (Pearce et al. 2009). Four socio-economic mobility trajectories were constructed (stable manual, stable non-manual, upward and downward). Retaining a functional dentition to age 50 was associated with social mobility among women only. Women in the stable non-manual group were most likely and women in the stable manual group were least likely to retain a functional dentition to age 50. Between ages 25 and 50, a gradient was apparent: no difference was observed between women in the stable non-manual and upwardly mobile groups, who were most likely to retain a functional dentition, followed by the downwardly mobile and then the stable manual groups. No associations were found between social mobility trajectories and oral health-related quality of life.

Evidence that social mobility influences oral health outcomes also came from the aforementioned study by Bernabé et al. (2011), who tested a social trajectories model using information on parental education at age seven and participants' own level of education in adulthood. The authors found that oral health among study participants became progressively worse across the following social trajectories and in that order: persistently high (high parental and high own education), upwardly mobile (low parental and high own education), downwardly mobile (high parental and low own education) and persistently low education.

However, analyses of the younger 1982 Pelotas birth cohort regarding the social trajectories model produced mixed findings. Family income trajectories between birth and age 15 were only partly associated with caries experience: adolescents who had been always poor had more decay and more unmet treatment need than those who had been never poor, but no differences were observed in these regards between upward or downward mobility and being always poor (Peres et al. 2007), suggesting that the experience of poverty, even if only at one stage in early life, was associated with poorer dental health. In a later study the same sample was followed up to age 24 years, thus including data from three time points (birth, age 15 and age 24) (Peres et al. 2011). This study reported a dose–response relationship between the cumulative exposure to poverty and the number of unsound teeth, supporting the accumulation of risk model. Participants who were socially mobile had better oral health than those who were poor at all three time points. No difference was observed between upward and downward social mobility, possibly because the observed time spans were too short for potential differences to play out.

Trajectories of Oral Disease

The team of researchers working on the Dunedin Multidisciplinary Health and Development Study have analysed trajectories of caries and dental plaque from childhood to young adulthood (ages 5–32), as well as periodontal disease between ages 26 and 38. The study follows all children born in 1 year (1972–1973) in the town of Dunedin, New Zealand. The initial sample comprised about 1,000 children, and the study achieved very good retention rates at later sweeps.

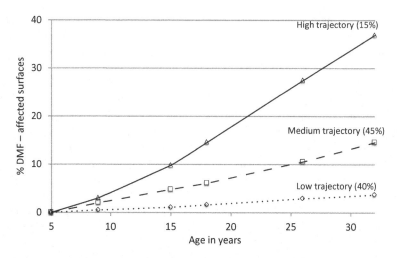

Fig. 3.5 Mean percentage of at-risk tooth surfaces affected by caries over time. Caries levels were measured at ages 5, 9, 15, 18, 26 and 32 (Reproduced from Broadbent et al. 2008)

Dental Caries

The progression of caries across the life course follows distinct patterns and trajectories, meaning that caries levels measured at one age predict caries levels at later ages. Broadbent et al. (2008) identified three distinct trajectories for the rate of increase in the percentage of caries-affected tooth surfaces in the permanent dentition, measured via the DMFS index (Decayed, Missing and Filled Surfaces) up to age 32. Of 955 participants who provided data at three or more time points, 40 % were in the low trajectory group, 45 % in the medium trajectory group and 15 % were classified as being in the high trajectory group. Interestingly, each of these trajectories was fairly linear, suggesting constant caries rates over time (Fig. 3.5). The authors concluded that although it is often assumed, there are no periods of markedly increased or decreased risk, and that therefore caries-preventive measures need to include all ages. However, longer follow-ups are needed to establish whether this is true also beyond the age of 32. The study was important in terms of describing caries progression patterns, but did not investigate which childhood and later life factors were associated with these different trajectories. Other research has consistently shown that caries in the primary dentition is a precursor of caries in permanent teeth (Sheiham and Sabbah 2010). The prevalence and severity of caries in the primary dentition are strongly related to individual as well as contextual socio-economic factors such as family income and maternal education (Hallett and O'Rourke 2003), as well as area deprivation (Locker 2000).

Dental Plaque

A separate study on the Dunedin sample investigated plaque levels over the same time period, as well as associations with caries, periodontal disease and tooth loss

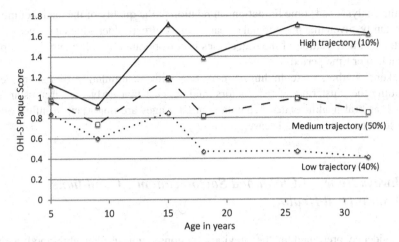

Fig. 3.6 Plaque trajectories by age. The graph shows the mean plaque levels for each trajectory group at ages 5, 9, 15, 18, 26 and 32 (Data source: Broadbent et al. 2011)

(Broadbent et al. 2011). Again, three trajectories were identified, with distributions that were strikingly similar to those found earlier for dental caries. Of 911 study participants, 40 % had plaque levels that were low and decreasing with age, 50 % had medium levels that were stable, and about 10 % had levels of plaque that were high and increasing (Fig. 3.6). Those in the high plaque group were more likely to be male, to have grown up in a family with a low socio-economic status, to have attained a lower level of education as adults, to be smokers and to be episodic rather than routine dental visitors. Allowing for the influence of childhood SES, sex, dental visiting patterns and smoking, plaque trajectories were strongly associated with caries experience, tooth loss and periodontal disease. The risk of periodontal disease was especially high among those who were smokers and had high levels of plaque at the same time.

Periodontal Disease

The most recent publication on disease trajectories coming from the Dunedin Study examined the prevalence and extent of periodontal disease through the ages 26, 32 and 38 (Thomson et al. 2013). The authors describe the following four trajectories for periodontal disease: very low (55.2 % of the sample), low (31.5 %), moderately increasing (10.7 %) and markedly increasing (2.5 %). Notable findings were a strong association between membership in the two "increasing" trajectories and long-term smoking, as well as a strong link between membership in the "markedly increasing" trajectory and low adult SES. The increase in periodontal disease was greater between ages 32 and 38 than it was between ages 26 and 32, which is to be expected as most periodontal disease occurs at later ages. The authors caution that the analysis had some limitations in relation to the quality of the data, but more importantly, given that periodontal disease mainly affects older adults it is necessary that the characterisation of the trajectories is corroborated by following the sample over a longer time period.

Taken together, these findings are in line with accumulation of risk models including the clustering of risk factors, and suggest that early life circumstances as well as oral health-related behaviours at later ages are important in influencing long-term patterns of oral disease.

Pathways Between Childhood Socio-economic Conditions and Adult Oral Health

The evidence presented in the previous sections suggests that childhood social conditions affect later adult oral health regardless of the socio-economic position that a person achieves later in life. But what are the pathways linking early circumstances and later oral health? The following sections describe some important findings in relation to potential mechanisms.

Early Malnutrition and Dental Caries

Early material disadvantage may result in malnutrition, a condition that is associated with deficiencies in protein, energy and micronutrients (Schroeder 2001). The links between early childhood malnutrition and dental caries have been discussed in a review by Psoter et al. (2005), who suggest two main mechanisms: via enamel hypoplasia and hypomineralisation (see also section "Developmental Defects of Enamel"), and via changes in salivary function, which include salivary flow, composition and buffering capacity.

An indirect marker of childhood malnutrition is stunted growth or height for age. The 1993 Pelotas birth cohort provided some longitudinal evidence for an independent relationship between height for age deficit at 12 months of age and higher caries levels at ages 6 and 12 years, after controlling for family SES (Peres et al. 2005, 2009). Similarly, in another Brazilian study taller adolescents had lower levels of caries experience in a sample of schoolchildren aged 15 (Freire et al. 2008).

Psychosocial Pathways and Oral Health-Related Behaviours

The link between childhood socio-economic status and adult health behaviours has been highlighted more than a decade ago in the highly influential work by Lynch et al. (1997). It is today widely accepted that social conditions in childhood influence educational attainment and adult life chances, and thereby shape peoples' psychological outlooks, such as their views about their futures and their feelings of control over their lives. Negative psychosocial dispositions, i.e. stronger beliefs in the influence of chance on health, and less thinking about the future are in turn related to health-compromising behaviours (Wardle and Steptoe 2003).

A psychosocial construct that is linked to people's sense of control and optimism is 'sense of coherence'. Sense of coherence is usually described as consisting of the three components comprehensibility, manageability, and meaningfulness in relation to one's internal and external environments (Antonovsky 1987). The role of sense of coherence in the relationship between parental education and adult oral health-related behaviours was investigated by Bernabé et al. (2009) in the Finnish Health 2000 Survey. The analysis revealed that parental education was indirectly associated with adult oral health-related behaviours, measured via a latent construct that included dental attendance, toothbrushing frequency, sugar intake frequency and daily smoking. The association was mainly mediated by adult socio-economic status measured via education and income, but to a lesser extent also by adult sense of coherence.

Support for psychosocial pathways comes also from two Brazilian studies which linked adverse family relationships, that is, high levels of paternal punishment and discipline, to the experience of traumatic dental injuries among adolescents (Nicolau et al. 2003), and also to periodontal disease among adult women (Nicolau et al. 2007a). Another study from Australia found that the recollection of a supportive parental rearing style was associated with more positive adult psychosocial attributes such as sense of control and satisfaction with life, which in turn was related to better subjective oral health (Sanders and Spencer 2005). But, all the studies mentioned here were cross-sectional and may have suffered from recall bias.

The biological mechanisms through which psychosocial adversity is translated into ill health have been investigated in a series of studies that examined the relationships between family financial stressors, oral cariogenic bacteria, salivary cortisol and dental caries among preschool children in the USA (Boyce et al. 2010). The researchers showed that dental caries was related to the number of cariogenic bacteria in the mouth, but there was a significant interaction: the association between caries levels and the number of cariogenic bacteria was stronger in children with high basal salivary cortisol secretion, which in turn was related to low family socio-economic position (Fig. 3.7). A possible explanation is that higher cortisol levels might affect immune competence and thus lower the defence against oral bacteria. This work provides evidence of a biological pathway that links higher levels of psychosocial stress with higher levels of caries in children.

Access to Dental Care

Data from the New Zealand Dunedin Study provided rare longitudinal evidence for the association between long-term dental visiting patterns and oral health (Thomson et al. 2010). The study followed participants between ages 15 and 32. After adjusting for SES and oral hygiene, those who were routine dental attenders, i.e. usually

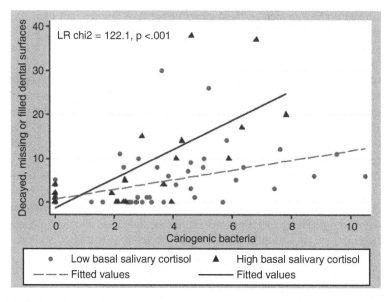

Fig. 3.7 Cariogenic bacteria and tooth decay, by level of cortisol secretion (Boyce et al. 2010)

visited the dentist for a check-up as opposed to visiting only when having a problem, had better oral health at any given age, and this effect was stronger the longer routine attendance was maintained. An association between retrospectively collected data on regular dental attendance since childhood and chewing ability at age 50 years was also reported in the study by Listl et al. (2014), based on the analysis of data from 13 European countries. These findings suggest that the relationship between routine dental visiting and better oral health is not merely due to a "healthy user" effect, but is indeed causal.

A Life Course Framework for Oral Health

The reviewed research has clearly shown that life course epidemiological models are very much applicable to oral diseases. Accumulation of risk including chains of risk, critical and sensitive period as well as social trajectories models are supported in the literature. Studying oral health from a life course perspective has provided insights into the importance of early life experiences, as well as lifelong trajectories of oral conditions. As is the case for general health, the underlying wider determinants of oral health are social. We therefore propose a theoretical framework for oral health that combines a life course perspective with the well-established models of the social determinants of oral diseases and their influence on the common risk factors that are shared between general and oral health (Fig. 3.8).

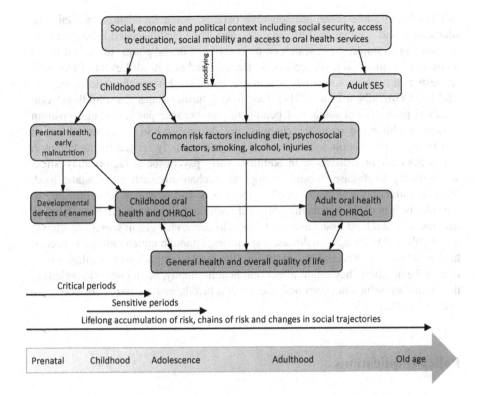

Fig. 3.8 A life course framework for oral health

The model emphasises the importance of socio-economic variables in childhood and adulthood such as education and income, which are influenced by economic, political and social factors at the societal level. This includes the degree to which childhood SES predicts adult SES, in other words the level of social mobility within a country, as well as national policies and provisions in relation to education, social security, public health and healthcare. One of the pathways through which early disadvantage might translate into poorer oral health is via developmental defects of enamel. The formation of dental enamel takes place within a specific time window, which for the primary dentition and some permanent teeth starts already in the womb. It has been shown that in line with a critical period model, stressors or disturbances during the development of enamel may result in irreversible defects, thus becoming embedded in the physical structure of the teeth (Seow 2013). Enamel defects that result in increased susceptibility to dental caries may be seen as part of a chain of risk (Psoter et al. 2005).

Another pathway is via the common risk factors that are known to affect oral as well as general health. In childhood, the main risk factors are a diet that is high in sugars, poor oral hygiene, and psychosocial stress, but also first experiences with tobacco and alcohol. Traumatic dental injuries are also socially patterned. Further, childhood and adolescence are sensitive periods, when foundations are laid for educational and occupational life chances, and when health-related behaviours are learned. For example, the research on trajectories of dental plaque discussed in the section on "Childhood Socio-economic Background and Adult Levels of Disease" suggests that hygiene habits adopted in childhood track through adolescence into adulthood (Broadbent et al. 2011). Our model further states that childhood oral health is predictive of adult oral health, in part because parental social position influences children's own life chances and destinations in terms of education and income, while adult social position is again strongly related to the common risk factors for oral diseases. In addition, early psychosocial factors may affect susceptibility to disease through biological mechanisms such as allostatic load. Further, childhood oral health directly influences oral health in later life, due to the colonisation of the oral cavity with oral bacteria and due to the irreversibility of damage to dental hard tissue and tooth loss. However, changes in social trajectories might still lead to changes in disease trajectories, although more evidence is needed to elucidate when such changes might have the greatest impact, how big they would need to be and how they might affect oral health. Finally, the model acknowledges the interrelationships between oral and general health, and the impact of both on a person's quality of life.

Policy Implications

The emerging evidence on the determinants of oral diseases from life course epidemiological studies has profound implications for future health and social policy. It is increasingly recognised that traditional preventive approaches which rely on clinical interventions and simplistic educational support are ineffective, costly and most likely increase oral health inequalities across the population (Watt 2005). Life course studies help to conceptualise how the social determinants of health influence oral health outcomes and in particular provide compelling evidence of the importance of early life factors.

Future oral health improvement strategies need to focus on addressing the shared underlying social determinants of chronic conditions, including oral diseases. Multi-strategy public health approaches are required which aim to create a supportive health promoting social environment conducive to good oral health and greater equity. Such an approach requires effective multi-sectoral working across a range of sectors, not just within the health care system. A particular priority is focusing on early life interventions to ensure that young children and families are given the best possible start in life. Public health interventions to promote health and well-being in early life need to utilise a range of complementary strategies including healthy public policy, creating supportive environments, strengthening community action, developing personal skills and ensuring evidence based support is provided by health and social care professionals. Although of fundamental importance, evidence on caries trajectories from adolescence to later adulthood highlight that getting a good start in life alone is not sufficient. Ongoing public health actions are also needed to protect and support good oral health across the life course. For example, oral health improvement strategies focusing on older people are needed to tackle high levels of disease amongst this group, and may also have important intergenerational effects.

Further research is needed to explore how oral health conditions such as enamel defects may be used as indicators of early life adverse exposures detrimental to health. Also, caries levels in preschool children are an accurate and relatively simple marker of social deprivation. Such approaches may help in targeting support to more vulnerable populations with particular needs.

Summary

Most of the research on oral health from a life course perspective has focused on the associations between childhood socio-economic circumstances and adult oral health. There is good evidence that early childhood is a sensitive period, influencing lifelong oral health trajectories. While the research suggests that the socio-economic conditions under which children grow up cast a long shadow on adult levels of oral disease, there is some evidence that these influences are amenable to change, however this area of research warrants further investigation.

Poor oral health is a marker of socio-economic disadvantage, and is strongly linked to general health. More research needs to be done to further our understanding of the interrelationships between oral and general health, and how they play out over the life course. A source of information that so far remains underused are developmental defects of enamel, which can provide a unique record of early life experiences.

While the prospective cohort study is the most desirable design to study life course influences on oral health, longitudinal studies that include clinical oral health data are very rare. So far, the available evidence rests mainly on three relatively small cohorts from England, New Zealand and Brazil. Reasons for this lack of data are likely to include costs, as the collection of clinical oral health outcomes by qualified dentists is expensive. Respondent burden might be another consideration. An alternative would be to use validated measures of self-reported outcomes such as self-rated oral health and oral health-related quality of life, which have been shown to correspond well with objective measures of disease (Pattussi et al. 2007). Unfortunately it is also quite likely that oral health is still seen as a low priority health outcome. We hope to have succeeded in highlighting the potential and importance of collecting high quality oral health data within cohort studies with large, nationally representative samples.

References

Antonovsky, A. (1987). *Unravelling the mystery of health: How people manage stress and stay well*. San Francisco: Jossey-Bass.

Azarpazhooh, A., & Leake, J. L. (2006). Systematic review of the association between respiratory diseases and oral health. *Journal of Periodontology, 77*(9), 1465–1482. doi:10.1902/jop.2006.060010.

Beaglehole, R., Benzian, H., Crail, J., & Mackay, J. (2009). *The oral health atlas. Mapping a neglected global health issue*. Brighton: FDI World Dental Federation.

Bedos, C., Brodeur, J. M., Arpin, S., & Nicolau, B. (2005). Dental caries experience: A two-generation study. *Journal of Dental Research, 84*(10), 931–936. doi:10.1177/154405910508401011.

Benjamin, R. M. (2010). Oral health: The silent epidemic. *Public Health Reports, 125*(2), 158–159.

Bernabé, E., Watt, R. G., Sheiham, A., Suominen-Taipale, A. L., Nordblad, A., Savolainen, J., et al. (2009). The influence of sense of coherence on the relationship between childhood socioeconomic status and adult oral health-related behaviours. *Community Dentistry and Oral Epidemiology, 37*(4), 357–365. doi:10.1111/j.1600-0528.2009.00483.x.

Bernabé, E., Suominen, A. L., Nordblad, A., Vehkalahti, M. M., Hausen, H., Knuuttila, M., et al. (2011). Education level and oral health in Finnish adults: Evidence from different lifecourse models. *Journal of Clinical Periodontology, 38*(1), 25–32. doi:10.1111/j.1600-051X.2010.01647.x.

Borgnakke, W. S., Ylostalo, P. V., Taylor, G. W., & Genco, R. J. (2013). Effect of periodontal disease on diabetes: Systematic review of epidemiologic observational evidence. *Journal of Periodontology, 84*(4 Suppl), S135–S152. doi:10.1902/jop.2013.1340013.

Boyce, W. T., Den Besten, P. K., Stamperdahl, J., Zhan, L., Jiang, Y., Adler, N. E., et al. (2010). Social inequalities in childhood dental caries: The convergent roles of stress, bacteria and disadvantage. *Social Science & Medicine, 71*(9), 1644–1652. doi:10.1016/j.socscimed.2010.07.045.

Broadbent, J. M., Thomson, W. M., & Poulton, R. (2008). Trajectory patterns of dental caries experience in the permanent dentition to the fourth decade of life. *Journal of Dental Research, 87*(1), 69–72. doi:10.1177/154405910808700112.

Broadbent, J. M., Thomson, W. M., Boyens, J. V., & Poulton, R. (2011). Dental plaque and oral health during the first 32 years of life. *The Journal of the American Dental Association, 142*(4), 415–426. doi:10.14219/jada.archive.2011.0197.

Cancer Research UK. (2012). *CancerStats key facts – Oral cancer*. London: Cancer Research UK.

Chaffee, B. W., Gansky, S. A., Weintraub, J. A., Featherstone, J. D. B., & Ramos-Gomez, F. J. (2014). Maternal oral bacterial levels predict early childhood caries development. *Journal of Dental Research, 93*(3), 238–244. doi:10.1177/0022034513517713.

Daly, B., Batchelor, P., Treasure, E. T., & Watt, R. G. (2013). *Essential dental public health* (2nd ed.). Oxford: Oxford University Press.

Dean, C. M. (2006). Tooth microstructure tracks the pace of human life-history evolution. *Proceedings of the Royal Society B: Biological Sciences, 273*(1603), 2799–2808. doi:10.1098/rspb.2006.3583.

Duijster, D., Sheiham, A., Hobdell, M. H., Itchon, G., & Monse, B. (2013). Associations between oral health-related impacts and rate of weight gain after extraction of pulpally involved teeth in underweight preschool Filipino children. *BMC Public Health, 13*, 533. doi:10.1186/1471-2458-13-533.

Freire, M. C., Sheiham, A., & Netuveli, G. (2008). Relationship between height and dental caries in adolescents. *Caries Research, 42*(2), 134–140. doi:10.1159/000121437.

Hallett, K. B., & O'Rourke, P. K. (2003). Social and behavioural determinants of early childhood caries. *Australian Dental Journal, 48*(1), 27–33. doi:10.1111/j.1834-7819.2003.tb00005.x.

Hobdell, M. H., Oliveira, E. R., Bautista, R., Myburgh, N. G., Narendran, S., & Johnson, N. W. (2003). Oral diseases and socio-economic status (SES). *British Dental Journal, 194*(2), 91–96. doi:10.1038/sj.bdj.4809882.

Holst, D., & Schuller, A. A. (2012). Oral health in a life-course: Birth-cohorts from 1929 to 2006 in Norway. *Community Dental Health, 29*(2), 134–143.

Humphrey, L. T., Dean, M. C., Jeffries, T. E., & Penn, M. (2008). Unlocking evidence of early diet from tooth enamel. *Proceedings of the National Academy of Sciences, 105*(19), 6834–6839. doi:10.1073/pnas.0711513105.

Jacobsen, P. E., Haubek, D., Henriksen, T. B., Østergaard, J. R., & Poulsen, S. (2014). Developmental enamel defects in children born preterm: A systematic review. *European Journal of Oral Sciences, 122*(1), 7–14. doi:10.1111/eos.12094.

Kramer, M. S., Séguin, L., Lydon, J., & Goulet, L. (2000). Socio-economic disparities in pregnancy outcome: Why do the poor fare so poorly? *Paediatric and Perinatal Epidemiology, 14*(3), 194–210. doi:10.1046/j.1365-3016.2000.00266.x.

Listl, S., Watt, R. G., & Tsakos, G. (2014). Early life conditions, adverse life events, and chewing ability at middle and later adulthood. *American Journal of Public Health*. doi:10.2105/AJPH.2014.301918.

Locker, D. (2000). Deprivation and oral health: A review. *Community Dentistry and Oral Epidemiology, 28*(3), 161–169. doi:10.1034/j.1600-0528.2000.280301.x.

Lynch, J. W., Kaplan, G. A., & Salonen, J. T. (1997). Why do poor people behave poorly? Variation in adult health behaviours and psychosocial characteristics by stages of the socioeconomic lifecourse. *Social Science & Medicine, 44*(6), 809–819. doi:10.1016/S0277-9536(96)00191-8.

Marcenes, W., Kassebaum, N. J., Bernabé, E., Flaxman, A., Naghavi, M., Lopez, A., et al. (2013). Global burden of oral conditions in 1990–2010: A systematic analysis. *Journal of Dental Research, 92*(7), 592–597. doi:10.1177/0022034513490168.

Marmot, M., & Bell, R. (2011). Social determinants and dental health. *Advances in Dental Research, 23*(2), 201–206. doi:10.1177/0022034511402079.

Mason, J., Pearce, M. S., Walls, A. W. G., Parker, L., & Steele, J. G. (2006). How do factors at different stages of the lifecourse contribute to oral-health-related quality of life in middle age for men and women? *Journal of Dental Research, 85*(3), 257–261. doi:10.1177/154405910608500310.

Needleman, H. L., Allred, E., Bellinger, D., Leviton, A., Rabinowitz, M., & Iverson, K. (1992). Antecedents and correlates of hypoplastic enamel defects of primary incisors. *Pediatric Dentistry, 14*(3), 158–166.

Nicolau, B., Marcenes, W., & Sheiham, A. (2003). The relationship between traumatic dental injuries and adolescents' development along the life course. *Community Dentistry and Oral Epidemiology, 31*(4), 306–313. doi:10.1034/j.1600-0528.2003.t01-1-00019.x.

Nicolau, B., Netuveli, G., Kim, J.-W. M., Sheiham, A., & Marcenes, W. (2007a). A life-course approach to assess psychosocial factors and periodontal disease. *Journal of Clinical Periodontology, 34*(10), 844–850. doi:10.1111/j.1600-051X.2007.01123.x.

Nicolau, B., Thomson, W. M., Steele, J. G., & Allison, P. J. (2007b). Life-course epidemiology: Concepts and theoretical models and its relevance to chronic oral conditions. *Community Dentistry and Oral Epidemiology, 35*(4), 241–249. doi:10.1111/j.1600-0528.2007.00332.x.

Pattussi, M. P., Olinto, M. T. A., Hardy, R., & Sheiham, A. (2007). Clinical, social and psychosocial factors associated with self-rated oral health in Brazilian adolescents. *Community Dentistry and Oral Epidemiology, 35*(5), 377–386. doi:10.1111/j.1600-0528.2006.00339.x.

Pearce, M. S., Steele, J. G., Mason, J., Walls, A. W. G., & Parker, L. (2004). Do circumstances in early life contribute to tooth retention in middle age? *Journal of Dental Research, 83*(7), 562–566. doi:10.1177/154405910408300710.

Pearce, M. S., Thomson, W. M., Walls, A. W. G., & Steele, J. G. (2009). Lifecourse socio-economic mobility and oral health in middle age. *Journal of Dental Research, 88*(10), 938–941. doi:10.1177/0022034509344524.

Peres, M. A., Latorre, M. R. D. O., Sheiham, A., Peres, K. G., Barros, F. C., Hernandez, P. G., et al. (2005). Social and biological early life influences on severity of dental caries in children aged 6 years. *Community Dentistry and Oral Epidemiology, 33*(1), 53–63. doi:10.1111/j.1600-0528.2004.00197.x.

Peres, M. A., Peres, K. G., de Barros, A. J. D., & Victora, C. G. (2007). The relation between family socioeconomic trajectories from childhood to adolescence and dental caries and associated oral behaviours. *Journal of Epidemiology and Community Health, 61*(2), 141–145. doi:10.1136/jech.2005.044818.

Peres, M. A., Barros, A. J., Peres, K. G., Araújo, C. L., & Menezes, A. M. (2009). Life course dental caries determinants and predictors in children aged 12 years: A population-based birth cohort. *Community Dentistry and Oral Epidemiology, 37*(2), 123–133. doi:10.1111/j.1600-0528.2009.00460.x.

Peres, M. A., Peres, K. G., Thomson, W. M., Broadbent, J. M., Gigante, D. P., & Horta, B. L. (2011). The influence of family income trajectories from birth to adulthood on adult oral health: Findings from the 1982 Pelotas birth cohort. *American Journal of Public Health, 101*(4), 730–736. doi:10.2105/AJPH.2009.184044.

Poulton, R., Caspi, A., Milne, B. J., Thomson, W. M., Taylor, A., Sears, M. R., et al. (2002). Association between children's experience of socioeconomic disadvantage and adult health: A life-course study. *The Lancet, 360*(9346), 1640–1645. doi:10.1016/S0140-6736(02)11602-3.

Psoter, W. J., Reid, B. C., & Katz, R. V. (2005). Malnutrition and dental caries: A review of the literature. *Caries Research, 39*(6), 441–447. doi:10.1159/000088178.

Reid, D. J., & Dean, M. C. (2006). Variation in modern human enamel formation times. *Journal of Human Evolution, 50*(3), 329–346. doi:10.1016/j.jhevol.2005.09.003.

Sanders, A. E., & Spencer, A. J. (2005). Childhood circumstances, psychosocial factors and the social impact of adult oral health. *Community Dentistry and Oral Epidemiology, 33*(5), 370–377. doi:10.1111/j.1600-0528.2005.00237.x.

Schroeder, D. (2001). Malnutrition. In R. Semba & M. Bloem (Eds.), *Nutrition and health in developing countries* (pp. 393–426). Totowa: Humana Press.

Seow, W. K. (1997). Effects of preterm birth on oral growth and development. *Australian Dental Journal, 42*(2), 85–91. doi:10.1111/j.1834-7819.1997.tb00102.x.

Seow, W. K. (2013). Developmental defects of enamel and dentine: Challenges for basic science research and clinical management. *Australian Dental Journal.* doi:10.1111/adj.12104.

Shearer, D. M., Thomson, W. M., Broadbent, J. M., & Poulton, R. (2011). Maternal oral health predicts their children's caries experience in adulthood. *Journal of Dental Research, 90*(5), 672–677. doi:10.1177/0022034510393349.

Sheiham, A. (2006). Dental caries affects body weight, growth and quality of life in pre-school children. *British Dental Journal, 201*(10), 625–626. doi:10.1038/sj.bdj.4814259.

Sheiham, A., & Sabbah, W. (2010). Using universal patterns of caries for planning and evaluating dental care. *Caries Research, 44*(2), 141–150. doi:10.1159/000308091.

Sheiham, A., & Watt, R. G. (2000). The common risk factor approach: A rational basis for promoting oral health. *Community Dentistry and Oral Epidemiology, 28*(6), 399–406. doi:10.1034/j.1600-0528.2000.028006399.x.

Sheiham, A., Alexander, D., Cohen, L., Marinho, V., Moysés, S., Petersen, P. E., et al. (2011). Global oral health inequalities: Task group – Implementation and delivery of oral health strategies. *Advances in Dental Research, 23*(2), 259–267. doi:10.1177/0022034511402084.

Sjögren, P., Nilsson, E., Forsell, M., Johansson, O., & Hoogstraate, J. (2008). A systematic review of the preventive effect of oral hygiene on pneumonia and respiratory tract infection in elderly people in hospitals and nursing homes: Effect estimates and methodological quality of randomized controlled trials. *Journal of the American Geriatrics Society, 56*(11), 2124–2130. doi:10.1111/j.1532-5415.2008.01926.x.

Thomson, W. M., Poulton, R., Milne, B. J., Caspi, A., Broughton, J. R., & Ayers, K. M. S. (2004). Socioeconomic inequalities in oral health in childhood and adulthood in a birth cohort. *Community Dentistry and Oral Epidemiology, 32*(5), 345–353. doi:10.1111/j.1600-0528.2004.00173.x.

Thomson, W. M., Williams, S. M., Broadbent, J. M., Poulton, R., & Locker, D. (2010). Long-term dental visiting patterns and adult oral health. *Journal of Dental Research, 89*(3), 307–311. doi:10.1177/0022034509356779.

Thomson, W. M., Shearer, D. M., Broadbent, J. M., Foster Page, L. A., & Poulton, R. (2013). The natural history of periodontal attachment loss during the third and fourth decades of life. *Journal of Clinical Periodontology, 40*(7), 672–680. doi:10.1111/jcpe.12108.

Tsakos, G., Herrick, K., Sheiham, A., & Watt, R. G. (2010). Edentulism and fruit and vegetable intake in low-income adults. *Journal of Dental Research, 89*(5), 462–467. doi:10.1177/0022034510363247.

UN. (2011). United Nations General Assembly. Political declaration of the high-level meeting of the General Assembly on the prevention and control of non-communicable diseases. Resolution. A/66/L1. 2011: Newyork

Wardle, J., & Steptoe, A. (2003). Socioeconomic differences in attitudes and beliefs about healthy lifestyles. *Journal of Epidemiology and Community Health, 57*(6), 440–443. doi:10.1136/jech.57.6.440.

Watt, R. G. (2005). Strategies and approaches in oral disease prevention and health promotion. *Bulletin of the World Health Organization, 83*, 711–718. doi:10.1590/S0042-96862005000900018.

Watt, R. G., & Sheiham, A. (2012). Integrating the common risk factor approach into a social determinants framework. *Community Dentistry and Oral Epidemiology, 40*(4), 289–296. doi:10.1111/j.1600-0528.2012.00680.x.

WHO. (2003). *Diet, nutrition and the prevention of chronic diseases*. Geneva: WHO.

Chapter 4
A Life Course Perspective on Body Size and Cardio-metabolic Health

William Johnson, Diana Kuh, and Rebecca Hardy

Introduction

During the twentieth century, populations around the world experienced an epidemiological transition, with morbidity and mortality increasingly being due to non-communicable diseases such as coronary heart disease (CHD) as opposed to communicable diseases such as influenza (Omran 1971). From a peak in the 1960s and 1970s rates of CHD have fallen in many of these countries, a fall which reflects both reduced incidence of disease and better treatment resulting in reduced case fatality rates (Beaglehole 1999). More recent analysis suggests that in England, CHD mortality has continued to decrease, although with variations by socioeconomic circumstances (Bajekal et al. 2013). Despite this fall, cardio-metabolic disease such as CHD, stroke, and type two diabetes, remain the leading cause of death in high income countries and are an increasing cause of morbidity and mortality in low and middle income countries (Yusuf et al. 2001). These diseases occur due to the impairment of an individual's cardiovascular system and/or metabolism and the risk of such diseases therefore reflects an individuals' cardio-metabolic health and thus measures of blood pressure, lipid, and glucose levels provide markers of cardio-metabolic health across the life course. The

W. Johnson (✉)
MRC Human Nutrition Research, Elsie Widdowson Laboratory, Cambridge, UK
e-mail: William.Johnson@mrc-hnr.cam.ac.uk

D. Kuh • R. Hardy
MRC Unit for Lifelong Health and Ageing at UCL, London, UK
e-mail: d.kuh@ucl.ac.uk; rebecca.hardy@ucl.ac.uk

© The Author(s) 2015
C. Burton-Jeangros et al. (eds.), *A Life Course Perspective on Health Trajectories and Transitions*, Life Course Research and Social Policies 4,
DOI 10.1007/978-3-319-20484-0_4

prevailing aetiological model for cardio-metabolic disease of the twentieth century emphasised adulthood risk factors because the diseases normally manifest for the first time in adulthood and are modifiable by lifestyle or environmental factors, such as diet, physical activity, and smoking.

Despite the dominance of the adult lifestyle model, there were a few initial reports suggesting that early life events might have long-term consequences for cardio-metabolic health in adulthood (Forsdahl 1977; Dorner et al. 1973; Dorner 1973; Freinkel 1980; Kermack et al. 2001). The study of Forsdahl (1977), for example, demonstrated a positive correlation between county level CHD mortality in Norway, in people aged between 40 and 69 years of age, and infant mortality 70 years earlier. It was postulated that poverty and food insecurity in childhood and adolescence were risk factors for CHD in adulthood. Finding a similar association between area level infant mortality and CHD mortality in the United Kingdom (UK), Professor David Barker from the University of Southampton hypothesised that environmental factors acting in utero or infancy may have adverse effects on CHD in later life (Barker and Osmond 1986). Direct evidence in support of this hypothesis was provided when Barker et al. (1989), linking individual birth records from the early decades of the twentieth century to subsequent mortality information, observed that the risk of death from CHD was greatest in individuals who were lightest at birth; birth weight being a conveniently available proxy marker of growth and nutrition in utero. A series of epidemiological studies followed seeking to confirm the initial birth weight-CHD association and extend it to include measures of postnatal growth and other health outcomes. The initial foetal origins of adult disease or programming hypothesis thus broadened, to become what is now known as the developmental origins of health and disease (DOHaD) model.

The importance of early life does not, however, mean that cardio-metabolic risk is set at the end of infancy and neither does it invalidate other models of disease causation. Indeed, at the same time that the DOHaD paradigm was developing, the term *life course epidemiology* was coined by scientists who recognised that disease development was more likely a lifelong process. They set out the key principles of this holistic approach in a series of papers and a book (Kuh et al. 2003, 2013; Ben-Shlomo and Kuh 2002; Kuh and Ben-Shlomo 2004; Kuh and Hardy 2002; Pickles et al. 2007; Lawlor and Mishra 2009; Koenen et al. 2013). Perhaps unsurprisingly, the role of body size in cardio-metabolic health played a central part in the development of the life course approach. The broad goal of this chapter is to synthesis this literature to better understand the lifelong age-related changes in body size that are indicative of poor cardio-metabolic health and the key environmental exposures and biological pathways responsible. We start with an overview of the life course approach in epidemiology to provide a framework for the review.

The Life Course Perspective

Definition

The life course approach to epidemiology focuses on investigation of the biological, behavioural, and social pathways (that may operate across generations) that link physical and social exposures and experiences during gestation, infancy, childhood, adolescence, and adulthood with health and disease risk in an individual (and possibly their descendants) (Ben-Shlomo and Kuh 2002; Kuh et al. 2003). Initially, the focus was on chronic degenerative diseases, particularly those pertaining to cardio-metabolic and respiratory systems, where the life course perspective was used to extend the DOHaD paradigm and integrate it with apparently conflicting theories of disease aetiology, namely adult lifestyle and social causation (Marmot et al. 1984; Krieger 2013). The life course approach then widened its gaze to a broader set of functional outcomes (e.g., grip strength and blood pressure) and emphasised the importance of age-related changes in physical and cognitive capability and the physiological systems on which they depend (Kuh et al. 2013).

From Conceptual Models to Trajectories

Conceptual models are a useful way to think about how an exposure measured across the life course may influence future health. The original conceptual life course models in epidemiology were developed to test the importance of timing and duration of exposures on disease risk (Ben-Shlomo and Kuh 2002; Kuh and Ben-Shlomo 2004; Kuh et al. 2003). The *critical or sensitive period model* depicts a scenario where some exposure has lifelong implications for disease risk, but only if (in the case of a critical period) or most strongly when (in the case of a sensitive period) that exposure occurs during some specific age window of development. The *accumulation of risk model* depicts a scenario where there is cumulative damage to biological systems due to multiple exposures over the life course, which may or may not cluster together. Finally, the *chain of risk model* depicts a scenario where an exposure at one age influences the likelihood of experiencing the same or a different exposure at a second age, and so on until the outcome occurs. If only the last exposure in the link influences disease risk, the model is said to include a trigger effect. Alternatively, if the exposures also have direct effects on the outcome that do not operate through subsequent exposures, the model is said to be additive. This can be thought of as a hybrid model comprising a chain of risk with some accumulation of risk.

These three types of model clearly do not capture the complexity of real life but they do provide a starting point for the conceptualisation of research questions, encourage consideration of duration, timing and order of exposures and aid effective communication of ideas. The initial emphasis in life course epidemiology had been in exploiting birth cohort studies to test what exposures measured across different periods of early life affected health and disease at a single time point in older age, but this emphasis is now moving toward gaining a better understanding of age-related disease processes and their life course determinants using the repeated measurements of health and function now available in many maturing cohort studies (Kuh et al. 2013). Such trajectories may themselves provide novel information on the disease process (e.g., how does blood pressure change over age?), maybe related to some future outcome (e.g., how are blood pressure trajectories related to CHD risk?) or concurrent process (how are blood pressure trajectories related to body weight trajectories?), or might themselves be the outcome (how is parental education associated with offspring blood pressure trajectories?). The statistical techniques needed to answer such questions are naturally becoming more and more advanced, and the reader wanting to learn more about methodology is directed to the following publications (De Stavola et al. 2006; Pickles et al. 2007; Tu et al. 2013; Johnson 2014).

Deleterious Body Size Trajectories

This section is split into life course stages. The summary compiles this information to discuss the lifelong age-related body size *trajectories* that are indicative of the worst cardio-metabolic health.

Gestation

Measurement of a baby at birth is the easiest way to assess the total growth experienced in gestation. In 1989, the first study to report on the relationship of birth weight with CHD was carried out in Hertfordshire, UK in 5,654 males born 1911–1930 (Barker et al. 1989). Standardised mortality ratios fell from 1.1 in men who weighed less than 2.5 kg to 0.8 in men who weighed more than 4.5 kg; a similar trend in women was subsequently reported (Osmond et al. 1993). Over the next few years, publications on UK studies established birth weight as also having a negative association with central obesity (Law et al. 1992), hypertension (Barker et al. 1990), stroke (Martyn et al. 1996), autoimmune thyroid disease (Phillips et al. 1993), chronic obstructive pulmonary disease (Barker et al. 1991), and type two diabetes (Hales et al. 1991) in adulthood. Ensuing work in the MRC National Survey of Health and Development of men and women born in Britain in 1946 found an inverse relationship of birth weight with blood pressure in midlife, as has been demonstrated in systematic reviews of available evidence (Huxley et al. 2002), but did not find higher birth weight to be strongly associated with a slower increase in blood pressure from 36 to 53 years (Hardy et al. 2003).

The birth weight-CHD association has now been replicated across multiple studies in Europe, North America, and South Asia (Stein et al. 1996). Many of the European studies demonstrated an association independent of confounding by gestational age and socioeconomic position. Nonetheless, the confounding structure has been widely debated in publications focusing largely on blood pressure (Hardy et al. 2006b; Huxley et al. 2002), as was the proposal that the negative associations may be a statistical artefact due to over-adjustment for adulthood body size (Tu et al. 2005). A potential reversal of the birth weight-blood pressure association from positive to negative on adjustment for adult size may occur because any relationship of birth weight with adulthood body mass index (BMI), a measure of weight standardised for height that is often used as an indicator of adiposity, is generally agreed to be positive not negative (Schellong et al. 2012). This is thought to be because birth weight is strongly predictive of later fat-free mass, arguably the largest component of BMI, and to a much lesser extent adiposity (Wells et al. 2007). From the start, there was also dispute about whether the relationships with birth weight, and particularly that for type two diabetes, were linear or U-shaped (Harder et al. 2007; Whincup et al. 2008).

Birth phenotypes other than birth weight identified as being associated with increased disease risk included short length, small head circumference, and low birth weight for placental weight (Barker et al. 1990, 1992, 1993), thereby suggesting that any form of growth restriction in utero has negative consequences. We do know from cohort comparison and famine studies, in which samples of pregnant mothers were exposed to chronic undernutrition, that brain tissue and adiposity are among the last body compartments to be affected (Yajnik et al. 2003; Z. Stein and Susser 1975). Compared to UK babies of healthy well-nourished mothers, for example, those born in rural India into a food insecure environment are smaller in all dimensions (−2.4 Z-scores for abdominal circumference), but least so for adiposity (−0.5 Z-scores for subscapular skinfold thickness) (Yajnik et al. 2003).

Infancy

The Hertfordshire Cohort Study also included health visitor records of weight at 1 year of age. Weight at this point in infancy actually had a stronger negative association with CHD than did weight at birth. Standardised mortality ratios fell from 1.1 in men who weighed less than 8.2 kg to 0.4 in men who weighed more than 12.2 kg (Barker et al. 1989). Infant weight also had a negative association with type two diabetes (Hales et al. 1991), but not with autoimmune thyroid disease (Phillips et al. 1993). The first publication to consider weight gain found that the greatest risk of CHD in men was in those born light who remained light at age 1 year, but in women was in those born light but who were heavy at age 1 year (Osmond et al. 1993); this sex difference was not discussed by the authors. Following studies generally found low weight gain and poor growth in infancy to be deleteriously associated with future cardio-metabolic outcomes (Eriksson et al. 2003b; Forsen et al. 2004). Today, rapid infant weight gain is known to be associated with obesity and obesity-related diseases (Kerkhof and Hokken-Koelega 2012; Druet et al. 2012). A recent meta-analysis of approximately 50,000 individuals in high income countries found that gaining weight between birth and age 1 year greater than one centile band on a growth chart was associated with a 23 % increased odds of adulthood obesity, for example (Druet et al. 2012). So, how does this not contradict the findings of the earlier studies? In those older cohorts, there would have been more environmental constraint on growth, thereby resulting in an at risk group who were born small and light and failed to catch-up in infancy with their better nourished peers. In the more recent studies, however, there would have been less constraint and more exposure to an obesogenic environment, thereby resulting in an at risk group who were not necessarily born small and light but nonetheless demonstrated rapid weight gain. Indeed, rapid infant weight gain is not necessarily deleterious if it occurs proportionally to increases in length (Belfort and Gillman 2013), and may even be protective in older cohorts and in low to middle income countries where it incurs gains in fat-free mass more so than adiposity (Wells et al. 2012; Bann et al. 2014).

The BMI is often used as a proxy for adiposity, despite never being intended for this purpose. Nonetheless, like percentage body fat, BMI shows a complex pattern of age-related change that can be summarised by the timing and magnitude of the maximum or peak value in infancy (Johnson et al. 2013b). Two studies have reported associations of both later timing and greater magnitude of this infant BMI peak with higher BMI later in life, one study in childhood (Silverwood et al. 2009) and one in adulthood (Sovio et al. 2014). In fully adjusted models in the latter study, a two standard deviation (SD) increase in age at peak was associated with a 1.58 % change in BMI at age 31 years and a two SD increase in magnitude of peak with a 4.65 % change. This finding is seemingly paradoxical to the observation of a secular trend toward earlier and lower peak as the environment has become more obesogenic (Johnson et al. 2013b). Changes in childhood BMI often reflect changes in fat-free mass more so than fat mass (Demerath et al. 2006), so it is not unreasonable to hypothesise that the positive infant peak-adulthood obesity association is driven by reduced fat-free mass in adults who experienced early and/or low peak. In agreement with the initial studies, the group of infants at risk has been proposed to comprise those with consistently low BMI in infancy (Rolland-Cachera and Peneau 2013).

Childhood

The BMI decreases in early childhood to a nadir named the adiposity rebound that occurs in most individuals between 5 and 7 years of age (Rolland-Cachera et al. 1984). Early occurrence of the rebound is associated with obesity and obesity-related diseases, even in the absence of elevated BMI at the age of rebound (Taylor et al. 2005), although this has been hotly debated in the past (Cole 2004). The most deleterious pattern is characterised by an early rebound and the crossing over of trajectory from low to high BMI (Rolland-Cachera and Peneau 2013). This pattern is in agreement with most secular trend studies (Johnson et al. 2012a), systematic reviews (Owen et al. 2009), and the initial studies (Barker et al. 2005). In the Helsinki Birth Cohort Study, for example, early rebound (less than 5 years of age) compared to late rebound (greater than 7 years of age) was associated with lower BMI in infancy, but higher BMI and cumulative incidence of type two diabetes (8.6 versus 1.8) in adulthood (Eriksson et al. 2003a). This crossing over of trajectory in children with an early rebound is driven by changes in adiposity rather than fat-free mass (Taylor et al. 2004). In contrast, the relationship of BMI at age 6 years to BMI at all previous and subsequent ages is driven by tracking of fat-free mass as well as adiposity (Rolland-Cachera and Peneau 2013). The rebound may, therefore, be a particularly important part of the establishment or otherwise of a deleterious trajectory (see section "Critical Periods and Transitions").

In addition to rapid weight gainers perhaps following an early rebound, there is likely to be a separate group whose poor growth persists in childhood (Cameron 2007). Both groups were identified as being at increased risk of hypertension in adulthood in the Helsinki Birth Cohort Study (Eriksson et al. 2007). Interestingly, the former trajectory had previously been reported to be associated with CHD (Barker et al. 2005), while the later had been reported to be associated with stroke (Osmond et al. 2007). Writing in a review paper, Barker et al. (2009) explains that the co-existence of these trajectories "casts light on the differing ecologies of CHD and stroke, for both of which hypertension is a risk factor". Rates of both CHD and childhood obesity, perhaps contributed to by rapid weight gain, increase as countries go through the epidemiological transition, but stroke remains most prevalent in low income countries where children tend to be short and thin.

Adolescence

Trajectories of children at risk carry forward so that in adolescence both high BMI/continued rapid weight gain and small body size/continued poor growth are associated with poorer cardio-metabolic health. Further, adolescence may be a particularly important stage in the life course for the establishment of a deleterious trajectory (see section "Definition"). A meta-analysis reported a positive association (relative risk 1.09, 95 % confidence interval 1.00–1.20) between BMI Z-score at 7–18 years of age and CHD (Owen et al. 2009). This and other meta-analyses tend to pool data across wide age ranges (Paajanen et al. 2010; Verbeeten et al. 2011) and estimates for the association of height specifically in adolescence with any cardio-metabolic health or disease outcome in adulthood cannot be found in systematic review literature. Most of our knowledge about the future health consequences of poor adolescent growth comes from stand-alone studies of historical birth cohorts and studies in low to middle income countries (Adair et al. 2013; Johnson et al. 2014; Skidmore et al. 2007). Greater height at age 15 years has been shown to be related to lower and thus more healthy total cholesterol and carotid intima-media thickness in the MRC National Survey of Health and Development, for example (Johnson et al. 2014; Skidmore et al. 2007).

The description of adolescents at risk becomes less clear when we consider the phenomenon that obese people tend to be temporarily taller than their non-obese peers by up to 3 cm in adolescence (Johnson et al. 2012b; Metcalf et al. 2011). This difference is similar to the temporary greater height of some girls compared to boys during adolescence, due to their earlier maturation (Ellison and Reiches 2012). The temporary greater height of some obese adolescents most likely reflects an advanced pace of development. Indeed, numerous studies in diverse populations have shown that adolescent obesity is linked to the earlier development of secondary sexual characteristics, most of which are in turn associated with shorter adulthood height (Dunger et al. 2005; Johnson et al. 2013a). Early timing of traits such as age at menarche has been implicated in cardio-metabolic disease processes (Prentice and Viner 2013; Hardy et al. 2006a), but whether or not they precede adolescent obesity or are causally related to adulthood disease independent of adolescent obesity remains unclear (Johnson et al. 2013a; Mumby et al. 2011; Pierce et al. 2012).

Adulthood

Linear growth is complete by adulthood, so the cardio-metabolic consequences of being short are less confounded by the constant change in ranking by height of individuals that occurs earlier in life. In one meta-analysis of data from over one million adults, a 6.5 cm increase in height was associated with a hazard ratio of 0.97 (95 % confidence interval 0.96–0.99) for all-cause mortality (Emerging Risk Factors Collaboration 2012). A body of literature has reported similar negative associations between adulthood height and other outcomes in diverse populations (Paajanen et al. 2010; Rosenberg et al. 2013; Schmidt et al. 2013). Further, we know that leg length, as a reflection of early life adversity (Wadsworth et al. 2002), is the main component of height associated with disease development (Langenberg et al. 2003; Wadsworth et al. 2002).

BMI in early adulthood has been shown to be associated with higher risk of subsequent CHD. The meta-analysis of Owen et al. reported a positive association between BMI Z-score between 18–30 years of age and CHD (relative risk 1.19, 95 % confidence interval 1.11–1.29) that was stronger than that in adolescence (Owen et al. 2009). Similar systematic reviews have been published for various cardio-metabolic biomarkers and diseases (Choi et al. 2013; Rao et al. 2011). Perhaps the most conclusive study of nearly one million adults reported a U-shaped association between BMI and all-cause mortality (Whitlock et al. 2009). Deaths in people with low BMI are most likely to be smoking and cancer related, whereas deaths in people with high BMI are most likely to be related to cardio-metabolic health (Whitlock et al. 2009).

Investigation is now focusing on whether those who were overweight in early life can alter their risk by being of normal weight in adulthood and whether duration of overweight is important. Literature has shown that obese children and adolescents who become normal weight in adulthood may have similar cardio-metabolic profiles as individuals who were always normal weight (Juonala et al. 2011; Li et al. 2012). Using data from the British birth cohort studies, however, Park et al. have reported higher odds ratios for type two diabetes in obese adults who were also overweight or obese in childhood and adolescence (odds ratio 12.6, 95 % confidence interval 6.6–24.0) compared to those who were obese in adulthood only (odds ratio 5.5, 95 % confidence interval 3.4–8.8), thereby suggesting that duration of exposure in addition to normalisation of weight status (i.e., change from obese/overweight to normal weight) is important (Park et al. 2013). One caveat here is that BMI tracks and increases across most of the life course, so the group who are obese in childhood and/or adolescence but normal weight in adulthood is typically small. Further, adults who are obese according to BMI may be metabolically healthy (Roberson et al. 2014). It has been hypothesized that it is this group of people who have consistently high BMI from infancy onward due to increased fat-free mass not adiposity (Rolland-Cachera and Peneau 2013). However, Ortega et al. have shown that a metabolically healthy obese group exists even when obesity is defined according to percentage body fat (Ortega et al. 2013).

Summary

The key traits associated with poor cardio-metabolic health in our literature review appear to naturally cluster into two groups. The first comprises microsomia in babies who despite being small are relatively adipose, postnatal growth failure particularly early in life, short adulthood stature and legs, and underweight or wasting/thinness at any age. Conversely, the second comprises macrosomia, rapid infant weight gain, early adiposity rebound followed by rapid BMI gain, tall stature in puberty, and peri-pubertal or adulthood obesity development. The first cluster characterises a trajectory of small size of most body dimensions and components (Fig. 4.1, Trajectory A) that might be found in older cohorts and studies in low income countries where there is constant persisting nutritional insecurity and high rates of stroke. Conversely, the second cluster characterises a trajectory of large size of most body dimensions and components (Fig. 4.1, Trajectory B), that might be found in modern day populations and high income countries where there are high rates of obesity and CHD. Most long-term follow-up studies have been conducted in cohorts that have experienced large changes in the environment over their life time or in studies in countries experiencing similar changes due to rapid nutritional and epidemiological transitions. It is perhaps, therefore, unsurprising that lying somewhere in between the first two trajectories is a third trajectory summarising this literature; it is characterised by small size and thinness at birth and in infancy, but rapid gains in weight and specifically adiposity in childhood, and the subsequent

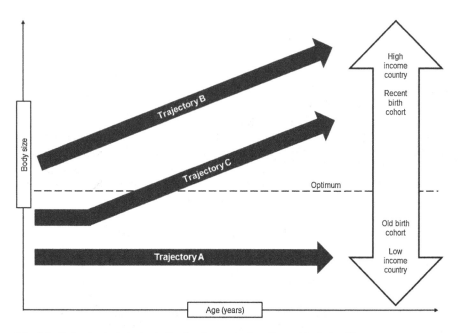

Fig. 4.1 Body size trajectories in the development of cardio-metabolic health

development of obesity and increased disease risk in response to the transitioning environment (Fig. 4.1, Trajectory C).

Clearly, the three trajectories in Fig. 4.1 are conceptual. While we split this section into life course stages for convenient handling of information, it is important to remember that each measure (e.g., weight and abdominal circumference) has its own trajectory that may follow a complex pattern of age-related change, demonstrate complex associations with cardio-metabolic health, and vary greatly between cohorts and across time, place, and population sub-groups. Further, traits in one trajectory might interact with traits in another trajectory to influence cardio-metabolic health. Considering birth weight and adulthood waist circumference, for example, risk for type two diabetes is greatest for individuals born light who went on to develop large waist lines (Tian et al. 2006).

Determinants and Mechanisms of Deleterious Trajectories

An association between body size at one age and cardio-metabolic health at a second age does not mean that the former causes the later. This section seeks to explain how and why body size across the life course may be associated with cardio-metabolic health.

Environmental Exposures

Foetal growth is ultimately restricted by uterine capacity. Babies may be born small because they are constrained in this way or because they lacked the nutrients in utero necessary for optimum growth (Harding 2001). Pregnant women exposed to famine give birth to small babies who go onto develop glucose intolerance and obesity in adulthood, for example (Ravelli et al. 1976, 1998). The proportion of protein and carbohydrate in a women's diet may be a key factor that affects the foetus, with the combination of high carbohydrate and low protein intake being particularly deleterious (Campbell et al. 1996; Godfrey et al. 1996). In addition to maternal intake per se, clinical exposures such as maternal hypertension leading to reduced uterine blood flow can severely affect the supply line of nutrients from the mother to the foetus (Harding 2001).

Other well-known determinants of size at birth include sex, gestational age, ethnic origin, parity, maternal and paternal size, gestational weight gain, general morbidity and episodic illness, malaria, cigarette smoking, and alcohol consumption (Kramer 1987). Maternal gestational diabetes is associated with higher birth weight and increased risk of subsequent obesity (Lawlor et al. 2011), but Gillman et al. (2003) have questioned the causal role of altered maternal-foetal glucose metabolism because adjusting the gestational diabetes-childhood obesity association for birth weight only marginally attenuated the estimate in their study. This might, however, be expected given that even the most exposed foetuses are limited to how much weight they can gain in utero; the greatest anatomical response to altered glucose metabolism will inevitably occur after birth, when there is no upper limit on weight gain. Indeed, the most deleterious profile for childhood obesity comprises rapid infant weight gain in addition to pre-pregnancy obesity and macroscomia (Weng et al. 2012).

Determinants of childhood obesity include maternal smoking, no or short duration of breastfeeding, obesity in infancy, short sleep duration, television viewing, low daily physical activity, and consumption of sugar-sweetened beverages (Monasta et al. 2010). Many of these risk factors continue to operate in adolescence (Morandi et al. 2012), at ages when there is increasing independence from the family and the establishment of more individual as compared to familial risk factors. Most research has focused on shifts in diet and physical activity as the key drivers of the obesity epidemic, particularly during adulthood (Swinburn et al. 2011; McAllister et al. 2009). There is, however increasing evidence for multiple other factors including microorganisms and epigenetics early in life, sleep debt, and endocrine disruptors (McAllister et al. 2009).

Naturally, the exposures responsible for obesity are very different to those for malnutrition. Evidence from low to middle income countries shows that the key determinants of stunting, wasting, and underweight include growth restriction in utero, poor condition of the mother, poverty, chronic dietary insufficiency, marked seasonality, poor levels of sanitation, and infection (Martorell and Young 2012; Frongillo et al. 1997). As these countries transition, it has been argued that the people are likely to face both sets of exposures and a dual burden of stunting and overweight (Varela-Silva et al. 2012). Others have, however, shown that the co-existence of stunting and overweight, at least at the family level, is a statistical artefact with a prevalence that matches what one would expect based on the separate stunting and overweight rates (Dieffenbach and Stein 2012).

Biological Pathways

Biological pathways are ultimately responsible for the links between environmental exposures, body size, and cardio-metabolic health. The first main type of pathway involves anatomical changes. Anatomical formation of the kidneys occurs exclusively in utero, and nutritional constraint of a foetus can permanently reduce the number of nephrons that are laid down, for example (Barker et al. 2006). Although physiological capability of the kidney develops over the entire life course, small kidney size in prenatally undernourished individuals increases risk for hypertension and renal failure in adulthood (Lampl et al. 2002; Luyckx and Brenner 2005). Similarly, a larger number of adipocytes in response to nutritional excess and a sedentary lifestyle in adulthood can increase CHD risk because these cells secrete inflammatory proteins that speed up the atherosclerotic process (Berg and Scherer 2005).

The second main type of pathway involves the physiological setting or alteration of hormonal and metabolic axes. For example, the foetus responds to reduced nutritional supply by reducing plasma concentrations of hormones, such as insulin and insulin-like growth factor, which in turn limits the transportation of glucose to the muscles and impairs lean tissue growth (Phillips 1996). This adaptation occurs so that glucose is readily available in the bloodstream to maintain growth of high priority organs, such as the brain (Gluckman 1995). The tendency to maintain high blood glucose levels can, however, lead to a progressive decline in glycaemic control and type two diabetes (Phillips 1996). As a different example, dysregulation of the hypothalamic-pituitary-adrenal axis in response to chronic stress in adulthood might lead through the effects of cortisol to central obesity and cardio-metabolic disease (Rosmond and Bjorntorp 2000).

One increasingly well-studied set of mechanisms focuses on the way in which genes governing body size impact on cardio-metabolic health. We know that environmental exposures can modify the expression of genes. A recent meta-analysis reported that the odds of obesity associated with the risk allele in the *FTO* gene was attenuated in active adults compared to inactive adults by 27 %, for example (Kilpelainen et al. 2011). Chemical modifications occur that alter gene expression in a specific tissue or organ without changing the nucleotide sequence of the DNA (e.g., methylation and histone modification) (Holliday 1994). While an environmental exposure may influence body size in the short term, these "epigenetic" changes can have long lasting effects on disease risk. Maternal protein restriction might lead to smaller offspring and reduce methylation (and therefore enhance expression) of the angiotensinogen receptor gene in the offspring adrenal gland, thereby leading to high blood pressure, for example (Bogdarina et al. 2007; Woodall et al. 1996). Such epigenetic changes can occur from conception onward but, like the other anatomical and physiological pathways, are most sensitive to the environment during specific stages of the life course.

Genes are also being used increasingly in Mendelian randomisation studies, where a genetic variant or set of variants are used as an instrumental variable for some phenotype or exposure, to establish whether or not that phenotype has a causal effect on some outcome (Lawlor et al. 2008). This technique has recently been used, for example, to demonstrate that BMI does have causal effects on various cardio-metabolic traits, including blood pressure and fasting glucose and cholesterol (Holmes et al. 2014). These studies work, subject to certain assumptions, on the premise that alleles are transmitted from parents to offspring randomly at gamete formation, such that the genotype or instrumental variable relationship with the outcome is not confounded by environmental factors or prone to reverse causation (Lawlor et al. 2008).

Critical Periods and Transitions

A critical period refers to an age window in which intrinsic changes in body structure and function are occurring rapidly and may be most easily programmed in a favourable or unfavourable direction (Scott 1986). The focus in the natural sciences was originally on the requirement of specific environmental stimuli to elicit the normal development and functioning of some body part or system (Cameron and Demerath 2002). In contrast, epidemiology focuses on the environmental exposures that result in anatomical and physiological adaptations that have long-term implications for cardio-metabolic health (Kuh et al. 2003). Perhaps the most often used example of a critical period is the teratogenic effect of maternal exposure to thalidomide in the first trimester of pregnancy on limb development in the foetus when the limbs are most rapidly developing, while exposure to thalidomide after birth is harmless (Newman 1986). In this instance, the critical period is truly critical. In other examples, however, the exposure association (with the outcome) is not constrained to such a narrow age window, but may be present across part or whole of the life course. The strongest associations are observed at ages when the individual is most sensitive to the environment, thus these are called sensitive periods of development.

Research has now identified potentially sensitive periods spanning the entire life course. Early childhood and adolescence in particular are emerging as important periods for the establishment of obesity and programming of cardio-metabolic risk. It has recently been shown in the MRC National Survey of Health and Development that socioeconomic disadvantage in early childhood, more so than at any other age, is associated with cardio-metabolic risk factors at age 53 years, for example (Murray et al. 2011). In the same cohort, exposure to obesity emerges during adolescence as being associated with greater carotid-intima media thickness at 60–64 years of age in men (Johnson et al. 2014). The associations reported in both of these papers were independent of birth weight and appeared to be mediated by higher adulthood BMI in those individuals who were disadvantaged in early childhood or obese in adolescence.

Adolescence is often viewed as critical from physical and behavioural perspectives, but individuals experience this stage in the life course at different ages and progress through secondary sexual characteristic maturation at different paces (Ellison and Reiches 2012). A critical or sensitive period may be thought of as a point of transition from one state to another. During puberty, for example, the adolescent transitions from an immature state to a mature state. Various markers of the pace of pubertal development have been reported to be associated with various cardio-metabolic health outcomes in both sexes (see section "Adolescence"). Interestingly, an early age at menopause, which marks the cessation of a women's reproductive ability, is also associated with increased risk for cardio-metabolic disease (Ebong et al. 2014). Lifelong environmental conditions may influence the timing of menopause (Lawlor et al. 2003), but it is unknown whether or not the biological changes that occur during menopause and impact on subsequent health are particularly sensitive to concurrent exposures. Similarly, behavioral transitions throughout the life course can lead to increased disease risk, but these do not necessarily occur at ages when biological changes are occurring rapidly and are most sensitive to the environment. Transition into a romantic relationship or marriage can cause behavioral changes that lead to the development of obesity (The and Gordon-Larsen 2009; Gordon-Larsen et al. 2004), but there is nothing biologically critical about the exact age when this occurs, for example. The same might be true for starting university (Gropper et al. 2012), leaving the army (Littman et al. 2013), and retiring (Morris et al. 1992). The timing of rapid change in a known biological structure/function is critical for the experience of specific environmental stimuli to cause permanent alterations and predict long-term outcomes (Cameron and Demerath 2002). While a critical or sensitive period may be thought of as a transition, a transition does not automatically meet the requirements to be a critical of sensitive period.

Transgenerational Transmission

Recent research in human and animal models suggests that biological adaptations to environmental exposures during critical or sensitive periods of development may be transmitted to subsequent generations (Benyshek 2013), such that a trait like insulin resistance in the exposed generation might be passed to successive unexposed generations in diminishing order of magnitude (Benyshek et al. 2006). This transgenerational transmission goes beyond something that might be explained by genetic heritability or by family members of different generations experiencing similar lifelong environments. Maternal exposure to famine, for example, has been shown to be associated with increased risk of giving birth to small offspring with dysregulated lipid profiles (Lumey et al. 2009), who themselves go onto have relatively small offspring with large amounts of adiposity and high risk for cardio-metabolic disease (Painter et al. 2008). In this scenario, direct and simultaneous exposure of three generations (i.e., the pregnant mother, her fetus, and the fetuses' primordial germ cells) might be responsible for the increased disease risk seen in each generation. Alternatively, and if more than three generations are affected, research is revealing how inheritance of epigenetic modifications to the genome may be responsible (Hackett et al. 2013).

Public Health Relevance and Conclusion

The role of life course research in public health debates, such as whether money should be spent on the primordial prevention of cardio-metabolic diseases in high risk strata of society or whether it should be used to provide effective treatment in the smaller number of people who actually develop a disease, is to provide clear empirical evidence of how and why a disease develops. Only then is it possible to understand what physical and social exposures should be targeted and at what ages. The conclusion of Barker et al. (1989) that "promotion of postnatal growth may be especially important in boys who weigh below 7.5 lb (3.4 kg) at birth" today may appear reckless. But this is only because a whole body of life course epidemiology literature has since been published showing that, at some ages and in some populations, rapid infant weight gain leads to the deleterious development of excess adiposity and may not incur protective long-term gains in height and fat-free mass (Bann et al. 2014; Druet et al. 2012; Kerkhof and Hokken-Koelega 2012; Wells et al. 2012). We may still not be at a situation where we should attempt to increase growth rates in infants who are born small, but we are developing a clearer picture of how, when, and in what populations this might be best achieved without adversely impacting on future health (Ong and Loos 2006).

Knowledge of the life course processes that lead to poor cardio-metabolic health and disease is relevant to many public health discussions and policies, not just those relating to infant growth and obesity. The life course perspective has become a central part of the World Health Organisation's programme on non-communicable disease prevention and health promotion (World Health Organisation Dept of Noncommunicable Disease Prevention and Health Promotion 2001). Particularly in the UK, the importance of a life course approach is increasingly gaining recognition, with recent reports on mental wellbeing and reproductive health having all championed the approach (Foresight. 2008; Scientific Advisory Committee 2011). The Marmot (2010) review on reducing health inequalities in the UK included statements, such as "giving every child the best start in life" and "enabling all children, young people, and adults to maximise their capabilities and have controls over their lives". The challenge life course epidemiologists now face is to fine-tune their studies to provide policy makers with the best, actionable information.

The literature on the relationships of body size with cardio-metabolic health is immense. Associations of body size with cardio-metabolic health can be explained in terms of anatomical and/or physiological changes in response to environmental conditions during critical or sensitive periods of development. These adaptations can persist across subsequent generations through epigenetic inheritance, thereby adding another layer of complexity to life course epidemiology. The integration of biological and social research is clearly important, as is the understanding of the processes and pathways operating across the life course. Taking this more holistic approach and understanding the life course trajectories of body size and cardio-metabolic health will lead to a more complete understanding of cardio-metabolic disease processes and how to stop disease processes progressing faster in some people than others.

References

Adair, L. S., Fall, C. H., Osmond, C., Stein, A. D., Martorell, R., Ramirez-Zea, M., et al. (2013). Associations of linear growth and relative weight gain during early life with adult health and human capital in countries of low and middle income: findings from five birth cohort studies. *Lancet, 382*(9891), 525–534.

Bajekal, M., Scholes, S., O'Flaherty, M., Raine, R., Norman, P., & Capewell, S. (2013). Unequal trends in coronary heart disease mortality by socioeconomic circumstances, England 1982-2006: An analytical study. *PloS One, 8*(3), e59608.

Bann, D., Wills, A., Cooper, R., Hardy, R., Aihie Sayer, A., Adams, J., et al. (2014). Birth weight and growth from infancy to late adolescence in relation to fat and lean mass in early old age: Findings from the MRC National Survey of Health and Development. *International Journal of Obesity, 38*(1), 69–75.

Barker, D. J., & Osmond, C. (1986). Infant mortality, childhood nutrition, and ischaemic heart disease in England and Wales. *Lancet, 1*(8489), 1077–1081.

Barker, D. J., Winter, P. D., Osmond, C., Margetts, B., & Simmonds, S. J. (1989). Weight in infancy and death from ischaemic heart disease. *Lancet, 2*(8663), 577–580.

Barker, D. J., Bull, A. R., Osmond, C., & Simmonds, S. J. (1990). Fetal and placental size and risk of hypertension in adult life. *British Medical Journal, 301*(6746), 259–262.

Barker, D. J., Godfrey, K. M., Fall, C., Osmond, C., Winter, P. D., & Shaheen, S. O. (1991). Relation of birth weight and childhood respiratory infection to adult lung function and death from chronic obstructive airways disease. *British Medical Journal, 303*(6804), 671–675.

Barker, D. J., Godfrey, K. M., Osmond, C., & Bull, A. (1992). The relation of fetal length, ponderal index and head circumference to blood pressure and the risk of hypertension in adult life. *Paediatric and Perinatal Epidemiology, 6*(1), 35–44.

Barker, D. J., Osmond, C., Simmonds, S. J., & Wield, G. A. (1993). The relation of small head circumference and thinness at birth to death from cardiovascular disease in adult life. *British Medical Journal, 306*(6875), 422–426.

Barker, D. J., Osmond, C., Forsen, T. J., Kajantie, E., & Eriksson, J. G. (2005). Trajectories of growth among children who have coronary events as adults. *New England Journal of Medicine, 353*(17), 1802–1809.

Barker, D. J., Bagby, S. P., & Hanson, M. A. (2006). Mechanisms of disease: In utero programming in the pathogenesis of hypertension. *Nature Clinical Practice Nephrology, 2*(12), 700–707.

Barker, D. J., Osmond, C., Kajantie, E., & Eriksson, J. G. (2009). Growth and chronic disease: Findings in the Helsinki Birth Cohort. *Annals of Human Biology, 36*(5), 445–458.

Beaglehole, R. (1999). International trends in coronary heart disease mortality and incidence rates. *Journal of Cardiovascular Risk, 6*(2), 63–68.

Belfort, M. B., & Gillman, M. W. (2013). Healthy infant growth: What are the trade-offs in the developed world? *Nestle Nutrition Institute Workshop Series, 71*, 171–184.

Ben-Shlomo, Y., & Kuh, D. (2002). A life course approach to chronic disease epidemiology: Conceptual models, empirical challenges and interdisciplinary perspectives. *International Journal of Epidemiology, 31*(2), 285–293.

Benyshek, D. C. (2013). The "early life" origins of obesity-related health disorders: New discoveries regarding the intergenerational transmission of developmentally programmed traits in the global cardiometabolic health crisis. *American Journal of Physical Anthropology, 152*(Suppl 57), 79–93.

Benyshek, D. C., Johnston, C. S., & Martin, J. F. (2006). Glucose metabolism is altered in the adequately-nourished grand-offspring (F3 generation) of rats malnourished during gestation and perinatal life. *Diabetologia, 49*(5), 1117–1119.

Berg, A. H., & Scherer, P. E. (2005). Adipose tissue, inflammation, and cardiovascular disease. *Circulation Research, 96*(9), 939–949.

Bogdarina, I., Welham, S., King, P. J., Burns, S. P., & Clark, A. J. (2007). Epigenetic modification of the renin-angiotensin system in the fetal programming of hypertension. *Circulation Research, 100*(4), 520–526.

Cameron, N. (2007). Growth patterns in adverse environments. *American Journal of Human Biology, 19*(5), 615–621.

Cameron, N., & Demerath, E. W. (2002). Critical periods in human growth and their relationship to diseases of aging. *American Journal of Physical Anthropology, 119*(Suppl 35), 159–184.

Campbell, D. M., Hall, M. H., Barker, D. J., Cross, J., Shiell, A. W., & Godfrey, K. M. (1996). Diet in pregnancy and the offspring's blood pressure 40 years later. *British Journal of Obstetrics and Gynaecology, 103*(3), 273–280.

Choi, J., Joseph, L., & Pilote, L. (2013). Obesity and C-reactive protein in various populations: A systematic review and meta-analysis. *Obesity Reviews, 14*(3), 232–244.

Cole, T. J. (2004). Children grow and horses race: Is the adiposity rebound a critical period for later obesity? *BMC Pediatrics, 4*, 6.

De Stavola, B. L., Nitsch, D., dos Santos Silva, I., McCormack, V., Hardy, R., Mann, V., et al. (2006). Statistical issues in life course epidemiology. *American Journal of Epidemiology, 163*(1), 84–96.

Demerath, E. W., Schubert, C. M., Maynard, L. M., Sun, S. S., Chumlea, W. C., Pickoff, A., et al. (2006). Do changes in body mass index percentile reflect changes in body composition in children? Data from the Fels Longitudinal Study. *Pediatrics, 117*(3), e487–e495.

Dieffenbach, S., & Stein, A. D. (2012). Stunted child/overweight mother pairs represent a statistical artifact, not a distinct entity. *Journal of Nutrition, 142*(4), 771–773.

Dorner, G. (1973). Possible significance of prenatal and-or perinatal nutrition for the pathogenesis of obesity. *Acta Biologica et Medica Germanica, 30*(5), K19–K22.

Dorner, G., Haller, H., & Leonhardt, W. (1973). Possible significance of pre- and or early postnatal nutrition in the pathogenesis of arteriosclerosis. *Acta Biologica et Medica Germanica, 31*(5), K31–K35.

Druet, C., Stettler, N., Sharp, S., Simmons, R. K., Cooper, C., Smith, G. D., et al. (2012). Prediction of childhood obesity by infancy weight gain: An individual-level meta-analysis. *Paediatric and Perinatal Epidemiology, 26*(1), 19–26.

Dunger, D. B., Ahmed, M. L., & Ong, K. K. (2005). Effects of obesity on growth and puberty. *Best Practice and Research Clinical Endocrinology and Metabolism, 19*(3), 375–390.

Ebong, I. A., Watson, K. E., Goff, D. C., Jr., Bluemke, D. A., Srikanthan, P., Horwich, T., et al. (2014). Age at menopause and incident heart failure: The Multi-Ethnic Study of Atherosclerosis. *Menopause, 21*(6), 585–591.

Ellison, P. T., & Reiches, M. W. (2012). Puberty. In N. Cameron & B. Bogin (Eds.), *Human growth and development* (2nd ed., pp. 81–107). London: Academic.

Emerging Risk Factors Collaboration. (2012). Adult height and the risk of cause-specific death and vascular morbidity in 1 million people: Individual participant meta-analysis. *International Journal of Epidemiology, 41*(5), 1419–1433.

Eriksson, J. G., Forsen, T., Tuomilehto, J., Osmond, C., & Barker, D. J. (2003a). Early adiposity rebound in childhood and risk of Type 2 diabetes in adult life. *Diabetologia, 46*(2), 190–194.

Eriksson, J. G., Forsen, T. J., Osmond, C., & Barker, D. J. (2003b). Pathways of infant and childhood growth that lead to type 2 diabetes. *Diabetes Care, 26*(11), 3006–3010.

Eriksson, J. G., Forsen, T. J., Kajantie, E., Osmond, C., & Barker, D. J. (2007). Childhood growth and hypertension in later life. *Hypertension, 49*(6), 1415–1421.

Foresight. (2008). *Foresight mental capital and wellbeing project. Final project report.* London: The Government Office for Science.

Forsdahl, A. (1977). Are poor living conditions in childhood and adolescence an important risk factor for arteriosclerotic heart disease? *British Journal of Preventive and Social Medicine, 31*(2), 91–95.

Forsen, T. J., Eriksson, J. G., Osmond, C., & Barker, D. J. (2004). The infant growth of boys who later develop coronary heart disease. *Annals of Medicine, 36*(5), 389–392.

Freinkel, N. (1980). Banting Lecture 1980. Of pregnancy and progeny. *Diabetes, 29*(12), 1023–1035.

Frongillo, E. A., Jr., de Onis, M., & Hanson, K. M. (1997). Socioeconomic and demographic factors are associated with worldwide patterns of stunting and wasting of children. *Journal of Nutrition, 127*(12), 2302–2309.

Gillman, M. W., Rifas-Shiman, S., Berkey, C. S., Field, A. E., & Colditz, G. A. (2003). Maternal gestational diabetes, birth weight, and adolescent obesity. *Pediatrics, 111*(3), e221–e226.

Gluckman, P. D. (1995). Clinical review 68: The endocrine regulation of fetal growth in late gestation: The role of insulin-like growth factors. *Journal of Clinical Endocrinology and Metabolism, 80*(4), 1047–1050.

Godfrey, K., Robinson, S., Barker, D. J., Osmond, C., & Cox, V. (1996). Maternal nutrition in early and late pregnancy in relation to placental and fetal growth. *British Medical Journal, 312*(7028), 410–414.

Gordon-Larsen, P., Adair, L. S., Nelson, M. C., & Popkin, B. M. (2004). Five-year obesity incidence in the transition period between adolescence and adulthood: The National Longitudinal Study of Adolescent Health. *American Journal of Clinical Nutrition, 80*(3), 569–575.

Gropper, S. S., Simmons, K. P., Connell, L. J., & Ulrich, P. V. (2012). Weight and body composition changes during the first three years of college. *Journal of Obesity, 2012*, 634048.

Hackett, J. A., Sengupta, R., Zylicz, J. J., Murakami, K., Lee, C., Down, T. A., et al. (2013). Germline DNA demethylation dynamics and imprint erasure through 5-hydroxymethylcytosine. *Science, 339*(6118), 448–452.

Hales, C. N., Barker, D. J., Clark, P. M., Cox, L. J., Fall, C., Osmond, C., et al. (1991). Fetal and infant growth and impaired glucose tolerance at age 64. *British Medical Journal, 303*(6809), 1019–1022.

Harder, T., Rodekamp, E., Schellong, K., Dudenhausen, J. W., & Plagemann, A. (2007). Birth weight and subsequent risk of type 2 diabetes: A meta-analysis. *American Journal of Epidemiology, 165*(8), 849–857.

Harding, J. E. (2001). The nutritional basis of the fetal origins of adult disease. *International Journal of Epidemiology, 30*(1), 15–23.

Hardy, R., Kuh, D., Langenberg, C., & Wadsworth, M. E. (2003). Birthweight, childhood social class, and change in adult blood pressure in the 1946 British birth cohort. *Lancet, 362*(9391), 1178–1183.

Hardy, R., Kuh, D., Whincup, P. H., & Wadsworth, M. E. (2006a). Age at puberty and adult blood pressure and body size in a British birth cohort study. *Journal of Hypertension, 24*(1), 59–66.

Hardy, R., Sovio, U., King, V. J., Skidmore, P. M., Helmsdal, G., Olsen, S. F., et al. (2006b). Birthweight and blood pressure in five European birth cohort studies: An investigation of confounding factors. *European Journal of Public Health, 16*(1), 21–30.

Holliday, R. (1994). Epigenetics: An overview. *Developmental Genetics, 15*(6), 453–457.

Holmes, M. V., Lange, L. A., Palmer, T., Lanktree, M. B., North, K. E., Almoguera, B., et al. (2014). Causal effects of body mass index on cardiometabolic traits and events: A Mendelian randomization analysis. *The American Journal of Human Genetics, 94*(2), 198–208.

Huxley, R., Neil, A., & Collins, R. (2002). Unravelling the fetal origins hypothesis: Is there really an inverse association between birthweight and subsequent blood pressure? *Lancet, 360*(9334), 659–665.

Johnson, W. (2014). Analytical strategies in human growth research. *American Journal of Human Biology, 27*, 69–83.

Johnson, W., Soloway, L. E., Erickson, D., Choh, A. C., Lee, M., Chumlea, W. C., et al. (2012a). A changing pattern of childhood BMI growth during the 20th century: 70 y of data from the Fels Longitudinal Study. *American Journal of Clinical Nutrition, 95*(5), 1136–1143.

Johnson, W., Stovitz, S. D., Choh, A. C., Czerwinski, S. A., Towne, B., & Demerath, E. W. (2012b). Patterns of linear growth and skeletal maturation from birth to 18 years of age in overweight young adults. *International Journal of Obesity, 36*(4), 535–541.

Johnson, W., Choh, A. C., Curran, J. E., Czerwinski, S. A., Bellis, C., Dyer, T. D., et al. (2013a). Genetic risk for earlier menarche also influences peripubertal body mass index. *American Journal of Physical Anthropology, 150*(1), 10–20.

Johnson, W., Choh, A. C., Lee, M., Towne, B., Czerwinski, S. A., & Demerath, E. W. (2013b). Characterization of the infant BMI peak: Sex differences, birth year cohort effects, association with concurrent adiposity, and heritability. *American Journal of Human Biology, 25*(3), 378–388.

Johnson, W., Kuh, D., Tikhonoff, V., Charakida, M., Woodside, J., Whincup, P., et al. (2014). Body mass index and height from infancy to adulthood and carotid intima-media thickness at 60 to 64 years in the 1946 British birth cohort study. *Arteriosclerosis, Thrombosis, and Vascular Biology, 34*(3), 654–660.

Juonala, M., Magnussen, C. G., Berenson, G. S., Venn, A., Burns, T. L., Sabin, M. A., et al. (2011). Childhood adiposity, adult adiposity, and cardiovascular risk factors. *New England Journal of Medicine, 365*(20), 1876–1885.

Kerkhof, G. F., & Hokken-Koelega, A. C. (2012). Rate of neonatal weight gain and effects on adult metabolic health. *Nature Reviews Endrocrinology, 8*(11), 689–692.

Kermack, W. O., McKendrick, A. G., & McKinlay, P. L. (2001). Death-rates in Great Britain and Sweden. Some general regularities and their significance. *International Journal of Epidemiology, 30*(4), 678–683.

Kilpelainen, T. O., Qi, L., Brage, S., Sharp, S. J., Sonestedt, E., Demerath, E., et al. (2011). Physical activity attenuates the influence of FTO variants on obesity risk: A meta-analysis of 218,166 adults and 19,268 children. *PLoS Medicine, 8*(11), e1001116.

Koenen, K. C., Rudenstine, S., Susser, E., & Galea, S. (2013). *A life course approach to mental disorders.* Oxford: Oxford University Press.

Kramer, M. S. (1987). Determinants of low birth weight: Methodological assessment and meta-analysis. *Bulletin of the World Health Organization, 65*(5), 663–737.

Krieger, N. (2013). *Epidemiology and the people's health: Theories and context.* New York: Oxford University Press.

Kuh, D., & Ben-Shlomo, Y. (2004). *A life course approach to chronic disease epidemiology* (2nd ed.). Oxford: Oxford University Press.

Kuh, D., & Hardy, R. (2002). *A life course approach to women's health.* Oxford: Oxford University Press.

Kuh, D., Ben-Shlomo, Y., Lynch, J., Hallqvist, J., & Power, C. (2003). Life course epidemiology. *Journal of Epidemiology and Community Health, 57*(10), 778–783.

Kuh, D., Cooper, R., Hardy, R., Richards, M., & Ben-Shlomo, Y. (2013). *A life course approach to healthy ageing*. Oxford: Oxford University Press.

Lampl, M., Kuzawa, C. W., & Jeanty, P. (2002). Infants thinner at birth exhibit smaller kidneys for their size in late gestation in a sample of fetuses with appropriate growth. *American Journal of Human Biology, 14*(3), 398–406.

Langenberg, C., Hardy, R., Kuh, D., & Wadsworth, M. E. (2003). Influence of height, leg and trunk length on pulse pressure, systolic and diastolic blood pressure. *Journal of Hypertension, 21*(3), 537–543.

Law, C. M., Barker, D. J., Osmond, C., Fall, C. H., & Simmonds, S. J. (1992). Early growth and abdominal fatness in adult life. *Journal of Epidemiology and Community Health, 46*(3), 184–186.

Lawlor, D. A., & Mishra, G. (2009). *Designing, analysing and understanding family based studies in life course epidemiology*. Oxford: Oxford University Press.

Lawlor, D. A., Ebrahim, S., & Smith, G. D. (2003). The association of socio-economic position across the life course and age at menopause: The British Women's Heart and Health Study. *BJOG, 110*(12), 1078–1087.

Lawlor, D. A., Harbord, R. M., Sterne, J. A., Timpson, N., & Davey Smith, G. (2008). Mendelian randomization: Using genes as instruments for making causal inferences in epidemiology. *Statistics in Medicine, 27*(8), 1133–1163.

Lawlor, D. A., Lichtenstein, P., & Langstrom, N. (2011). Association of maternal diabetes mellitus in pregnancy with offspring adiposity into early adulthood: Sibling study in a prospective cohort of 280,866 men from 248,293 families. *Circulation, 123*(3), 258–265.

Li, S., Chen, W., Srinivasan, S. R., Xu, J., & Berenson, G. S. (2012). Relation of childhood obesity/cardiometabolic phenotypes to adult cardiometabolic profile: The Bogalusa Heart Study. *American Journal of Epidemiology, 176*(Suppl 7), S142–S149.

Littman, A. J., Jacobson, I. G., Boyko, E. J., Powell, T. M., & Smith, T. C. (2013). Weight change following US military service. *International Journal of Obesity, 37*(2), 244–253.

Lumey, L. H., Stein, A. D., Kahn, H. S., & Romijn, J. A. (2009). Lipid profiles in middle-aged men and women after famine exposure during gestation: The Dutch Hunger Winter Families Study. *American Journal of Clinical Nutrition, 89*(6), 1737–1743.

Luyckx, V. A., & Brenner, B. M. (2005). Low birth weight, nephron number, and kidney disease. *Kidney International Supplement, 68*(97), S68–S77.

Marmot, M. G. (2010). *Fair society, healthy lives: The Marmot review*. London: UCL Institute of Health Equity.

Marmot, M. G., Shipley, M. J., & Rose, G. (1984). Inequalities in death–specific explanations of a general pattern? *Lancet, 1*(8384), 1003–1006.

Martorell, R., & Young, M. F. (2012). Patterns of stunting and wasting: Potential explanatory factors. *Advances in Nutrition, 3*(2), 227–233.

Martyn, C. N., Barker, D. J., & Osmond, C. (1996). Mothers' pelvic size, fetal growth, and death from stroke and coronary heart disease in men in the UK. *Lancet, 348*(9037), 1264–1268.

McAllister, E. J., Dhurandhar, N. V., Keith, S. W., Aronne, L. J., Barger, J., Baskin, M., et al. (2009). Ten putative contributors to the obesity epidemic. *Critical Reviews in Food Science and Nutrition, 49*(10), 868–913.

Metcalf, B. S., Hosking, J., Fremeaux, A. E., Jeffery, A. N., Voss, L. D., & Wilkin, T. J. (2011). BMI was right all along: Taller children really are fatter (implications of making childhood BMI independent of height) EarlyBird 48. *International Journal of Obesity, 35*(4), 541–547.

Monasta, L., Batty, G. D., Cattaneo, A., Lutje, V., Ronfani, L., Van Lenthe, F. J., et al. (2010). Early-life determinants of overweight and obesity: A review of systematic reviews. *Obesity Reviews, 11*(10), 695–708.

Morandi, A., Meyre, D., Lobbens, S., Kleinman, K., Kaakinen, M., Rifas-Shiman, S. L., et al. (2012). Estimation of newborn risk for child or adolescent obesity: Lessons from longitudinal birth cohorts. *PloS One, 7*(11), e49919.

Morris, J. K., Cook, D. G., & Shaper, A. G. (1992). Non-employment and changes in smoking, drinking, and body weight. *British Medical Journal, 304*(6826), 536–541.

Mumby, H. S., Elks, C. E., Li, S., Sharp, S. J., Khaw, K. T., Luben, R. N., et al. (2011). Mendelian Randomisation Study of Childhood BMI and Early Menarche. *Journal of Obesity, 2011*, 180729.

Murray, E. T., Mishra, G. D., Kuh, D., Guralnik, J., Black, S., & Hardy, R. (2011). Life course models of socioeconomic position and cardiovascular risk factors: 1946 birth cohort. *Annals of Epidemiology, 21*(8), 589–597.

Newman, C. G. (1986). The thalidomide syndrome: Risks of exposure and spectrum of malformations. *Clinics in Perinatology, 13*(3), 555–573.

Omran, A. R. (1971). The epidemiologic transition. A theory of the epidemiology of population change. *Milbank Memorial Fund Quarterly, 49*(4), 509–538.

Ong, K. K., & Loos, R. J. (2006). Rapid infancy weight gain and subsequent obesity: Systematic reviews and hopeful suggestions. *Acta Paediatrica, 95*(8), 904–908.

Ortega, F. B., Lee, D. C., Katzmarzyk, P. T., Ruiz, J. R., Sui, X., Church, T. S., et al. (2013). The intriguing metabolically healthy but obese phenotype: Cardiovascular prognosis and role of fitness. *European Heart Journal, 34*(5), 389–397.

Osmond, C., Barker, D. J., Winter, P. D., Fall, C. H., & Simmonds, S. J. (1993). Early growth and death from cardiovascular disease in women. *British Medical Journal, 307*(6918), 1519–1524.

Osmond, C., Kajantie, E., Forsen, T. J., Eriksson, J. G., & Barker, D. J. (2007). Infant growth and stroke in adult life: The Helsinki birth cohort study. *Stroke, 38*(2), 264–270.

Owen, C. G., Whincup, P. H., Orfei, L., Chou, Q. A., Rudnicka, A. R., Wathern, A. K., et al. (2009). Is body mass index before middle age related to coronary heart disease risk in later life? Evidence from observational studies. *International Journal of Obesity, 33*(8), 866–877.

Paajanen, T. A., Oksala, N. K., Kuukasjarvi, P., & Karhunen, P. J. (2010). Short stature is associated with coronary heart disease: A systematic review of the literature and a meta-analysis. *European Heart Journal, 31*(14), 1802–1809.

Painter, R. C., Osmond, C., Gluckman, P., Hanson, M., Phillips, D. I., & Roseboom, T. J. (2008). Transgenerational effects of prenatal exposure to the Dutch famine on neonatal adiposity and health in later life. *BJOG, 115*(10), 1243–1249.

Park, M. H., Sovio, U., Viner, R. M., Hardy, R. J., & Kinra, S. (2013). Overweight in childhood, adolescence and adulthood and cardiovascular risk in later life: Pooled analysis of three British birth cohorts. *PloS One, 8*(7), e70684.

Phillips, D. I. (1996). Insulin resistance as a programmed response to fetal undernutrition. *Diabetologia, 39*(9), 1119–1122.

Phillips, D. I., Cooper, C., Fall, C., Prentice, L., Osmond, C., Barker, D. J., et al. (1993). Fetal growth and autoimmune thyroid disease. *Quarterly Journal of Medicine, 86*(4), 247–253.

Pickles, A., Maughan, B., & Wadsworth, M. (2007). *Epidemiological methods in life course research.* Oxford: Oxford University Press.

Pierce, M. B., Kuh, D., & Hardy, R. (2012). The role of BMI across the life course in the relationship between age at menarche and diabetes, in a British Birth Cohort. *Diabetic Medicine, 29*(5), 600–603.

Prentice, P., & Viner, R. M. (2013). Pubertal timing and adult obesity and cardiometabolic risk in women and men: A systematic review and meta-analysis. *International Journal of Obesity, 37*(8), 1036–1043.

Rao, G. H., Thethi, I., & Fareed, J. (2011). Vascular disease: Obesity and excess weight as modulators of risk. *Expert Review of Cardiovascular Therapy, 9*(4), 525–534.

Ravelli, G. P., Stein, Z. A., & Susser, M. W. (1976). Obesity in young men after famine exposure in utero and early infancy. *New England Journal of Medicine, 295*(7), 349–353.

Ravelli, A. C., van der Meulen, J. H., Michels, R. P., Osmond, C., Barker, D. J., Hales, C. N., et al. (1998). Glucose tolerance in adults after prenatal exposure to famine. *Lancet, 351*(9097), 173–177.

Roberson, L. L., Aneni, E. C., Maziak, W., Agatston, A., Feldman, T., Rouseff, M., et al. (2014). Beyond BMI: The "Metabolically healthy obese" phenotype & its association with clinical/subclinical cardiovascular disease and all-cause mortality – a systematic review. *BMC Public Health, 14*(1), 14.

Rolland-Cachera, M. F., & Peneau, S. (2013). Growth trajectories associated with adult obesity. *World Review of Nutrition and Dietetics, 106*, 127–134.

Rolland-Cachera, M. F., Deheeger, M., Bellisle, F., Sempe, M., Guilloud-Bataille, M., & Patois, E. (1984). Adiposity rebound in children: A simple indicator for predicting obesity. *American Journal of Clinical Nutrition, 39*(1), 129–135.

Rosenberg, M. A., Lopez, F. L., Buzkova, P., Adabag, S., Chen, L. Y., Sotoodehnia, N., et al. (2013). Height and risk of sudden cardiac death: The Atherosclerosis Risk in Communities and Cardiovascular Health Studies. *Annals of Epidemiology, 24*(3), 174–179.

Rosmond, R., & Bjorntorp, P. (2000). The hypothalamic-pituitary-adrenal axis activity as a predictor of cardiovascular disease, type 2 diabetes and stroke. *Journal of Internal Medicine, 247*(2), 188–197.

Schellong, K., Schulz, S., Harder, T., & Plagemann, A. (2012). Birth weight and long-term overweight risk: Systematic review and a meta-analysis including 643,902 persons from 66 studies and 26 countries globally. *PloS One, 7*(10), e47776.

Schmidt, M., Botker, H. E., Pedersen, L., & Sorensen, H. T. (2013). Adult height and risk of ischemic heart disease, atrial fibrillation, stroke, venous thromboembolism, and premature death: A population based 36-year follow-up study. *European Journal of Epidemiology, 29*(2), 111–118.

Scientific Advisory Committee. (2011). *Opinion paper 27: Why should we consider a life course approach to women's health care*. London: Royal College of Obstetricians and Gynaecologists.

Scott, J. P. (1986). Critical periods in organizational processes. In F. Falkner & J. M. Tanner (Eds.), *Human growth: A comprehensive treatise* (Methodology; ecological, genetic and nutritional effects on growth, Vol. 3, pp. 181–196). New York: Plenum Press.

Silverwood, R. J., De Stavola, B. L., Cole, T. J., & Leon, D. A. (2009). BMI peak in infancy as a predictor for later BMI in the Uppsala Family Study. *International Journal of Obesity, 33*(8), 929–937.

Skidmore, P. M., Hardy, R. J., Kuh, D. J., Langenberg, C., & Wadsworth, M. E. (2007). Life course body size and lipid levels at 53 years in a British birth cohort. *Journal of Epidemiology and Community Health, 61*(3), 215–220.

Sovio, U., Kaakinen, M., Tzoulaki, I., Das, S., Ruokonen, A., Pouta, A., et al. (2014). How do changes in body mass index in infancy and childhood associate with cardiometabolic profile in adulthood? Findings from the Northern Finland Birth Cohort 1966 Study. *International Journal of Obesity, 38*(1), 53–59.

Stein, Z., & Susser, M. (1975). The Dutch famine, 1944-1945, and the reproductive process. I. Effects on six indices at birth. *Pediatric Research, 9*(2), 70–76.

Stein, C. E., Fall, C. H., Kumaran, K., Osmond, C., Cox, V., & Barker, D. J. (1996). Fetal growth and coronary heart disease in south India. *Lancet, 348*(9037), 1269–1273.

Swinburn, B. A., Sacks, G., Hall, K. D., McPherson, K., Finegood, D. T., Moodie, M. L., et al. (2011). The global obesity pandemic: Shaped by global drivers and local environments. *Lancet, 378*(9793), 804–814.

Taylor, R. W., Goulding, A., Lewis-Barned, N. J., & Williams, S. M. (2004). Rate of fat gain is faster in girls undergoing early adiposity rebound. *Obesity Research, 12*(8), 1228–1230.

Taylor, R. W., Grant, A. M., Goulding, A., & Williams, S. M. (2005). Early adiposity rebound: Review of papers linking this to subsequent obesity in children and adults. *Current Opinion in Clinical Nutrition and Metabolic Care, 8*(6), 607–612.

The, N. S., & Gordon-Larsen, P. (2009). Entry into romantic partnership is associated with obesity. *Obesity (Silver Spring), 17*(7), 1441–1447.

Tian, J. Y., Cheng, Q., Song, X. M., Li, G., Jiang, G. X., Gu, Y. Y., et al. (2006). Birth weight and risk of type 2 diabetes, abdominal obesity and hypertension among Chinese adults. *European Journal of Endocrinology, 155*(4), 601–607.

Tu, Y. K., West, R., Ellison, G. T., & Gilthorpe, M. S. (2005). Why evidence for the fetal origins of adult disease might be a statistical artifact: The "reversal paradox" for the relation between birth weight and blood pressure in later life. *American Journal of Epidemiology, 161*(1), 27–32.

Tu, Y. K., Tilling, K., Sterne, J. A., & Gilthorpe, M. S. (2013). A critical evaluation of statistical approaches to examining the role of growth trajectories in the developmental origins of health and disease. *International Journal of Epidemiology, 42*(5), 1327–1339.

Varela-Silva, M. I., Dickinson, F., Wilson, H., Azcorra, H., Griffiths, P. L., & Bogin, B. (2012). The nutritional dual-burden in developing countries–how is it assessed and what are the health implications? *Collegium Antropologicum, 36*(1), 39–45.

Verbeeten, K. C., Elks, C. E., Daneman, D., & Ong, K. K. (2011). Association between childhood obesity and subsequent Type 1 diabetes: A systematic review and meta-analysis. *Diabetic Medicine, 28*(1), 10–18.

Wadsworth, M. E., Hardy, R. J., Paul, A. A., Marshall, S. F., & Cole, T. J. (2002). Leg and trunk length at 43 years in relation to childhood health, diet and family circumstances; evidence from the 1946 national birth cohort. *International Journal of Epidemiology, 31*(2), 383–390.

Wells, J. C., Chomtho, S., & Fewtrell, M. S. (2007). Programming of body composition by early growth and nutrition. *Proceedings of the Nutrition Society, 66*(3), 423–434.

Wells, J. C., Dumith, S. C., Ekelund, U., Reichert, F. F., Menezes, A. M., Victora, C. G., et al. (2012). Associations of intrauterine and postnatal weight and length gains with adolescent body composition: Prospective birth cohort study from Brazil. *Journal of Adolescent Health, 51*(6 Suppl), S58–S64.

Weng, S. F., Redsell, S. A., Swift, J. A., Yang, M., & Glazebrook, C. P. (2012). Systematic review and meta-analyses of risk factors for childhood overweight identifiable during infancy. *Archives of Disease in Childhood, 97*(12), 1019–1026.

Whincup, P. H., Kaye, S. J., Owen, C. G., Huxley, R., Cook, D. G., Anazawa, S., et al. (2008). Birth weight and risk of type 2 diabetes: A systematic review. *Journal of the American Medical Association, 300*(24), 2886–2897.

Whitlock, G., Lewington, S., Sherliker, P., Clarke, R., Emberson, J., Halsey, J., et al. (2009). Body-mass index and cause-specific mortality in 900 000 adults: Collaborative analyses of 57 prospective studies. *Lancet, 373*(9669), 1083–1096.

Woodall, S. M., Johnston, B. M., Breier, B. H., & Gluckman, P. D. (1996). Chronic maternal undernutrition in the rat leads to delayed postnatal growth and elevated blood pressure of offspring. *Pediatric Research, 40*(3), 438–443.

Yajnik, C. S., Fall, C. H., Coyaji, K. J., Hirve, S. S., Rao, S., Barker, D. J., et al. (2003). Neonatal anthropometry: The thin-fat Indian baby. The Pune Maternal Nutrition Study. *International Journal of Obesity, 27*(2), 173–180.

Yusuf, S., Reddy, S., Ounpuu, S., & Anand, S. (2001). Global burden of cardiovascular diseases: Part I: General considerations, the epidemiologic transition, risk factors, and impact of urbanization. *Circulation, 104*(22), 2746–2753.

World Health Organisation Department of Noncommunicable Disease Prevention and Health Promotion. (2001). Life course perspectives on coronary heart disease, stroke and diabetes: Key issues and implications for policy and research: Summary report of a meeting of experts, 2–4 May 2001. Geneva: World Health Organisation.

Chapter 5
Health Trajectories in People with Cystic Fibrosis in the UK: Exploring the Effect of Social Deprivation

David Taylor-Robinson, Peter Diggle, Rosalind Smyth, and Margaret Whitehead

Cystic Fibrosis As a Case for Studying Health Inequalities

Exploring the reasons for inequalities in outcomes in people with cystic fibrosis (CF) offers a unique opportunity to develop our understanding around pathways in inequalities in health more generally. Because CF is genetically determined, a socio-economic difference in incidence is not expected, but there may be important differences in outcomes over the course of people's lives.

Studies across the world have consistently shown that people from socio-economically disadvantaged backgrounds experience worse health than those in more socio-economically advantaged positions. These inequalities in health outcomes are preventable, amenable to policy intervention, and they are unjust. In the UK and internationally, policies are being implemented to try to reduce health inequalities, with limited success, since for many important health outcomes, such as life expectancy in the UK, despite continuing overall improvements, significant inequalities remain (Marmot et al. 2010; Barr et al. 2012). In order to develop more effective interventions, we need a better understanding of how, and when, these health differences are generated and maintained.

This chapter brings together findings from our previously published longitudinal registry studies examining the effect of social deprivation on longitudinal clinical outcomes, healthcare use and employment opportunities in people with cystic

D. Taylor-Robinson (✉) • P. Diggle • M. Whitehead
University of Liverpool, Liverpool, UK
e-mail: David.Taylor-Robinson@liverpool.ac.uk; P.Diggle@liverpool.ac.uk; Mmw@liverpool.ac.uk

R. Smyth
UCL, London, UK
e-mail: rosalind.smyth@ucl.ac.uk

© The Author(s) 2015
C. Burton-Jeangros et al. (eds.), *A Life Course Perspective on Health Trajectories and Transitions*, Life Course Research and Social Policies 4,
DOI 10.1007/978-3-319-20484-0_5

fibrosis (CF), and draws on material from the lead author's PhD thesis, from which some sections are reproduced (Taylor-Robinson 2013; Taylor-Robinson et al. 2013a, b). Studying the health of people with CF in this way provides a valuable case study to investigate the impact of social deprivation on health and social outcomes, in a chronic condition *without a socio-economic gradient in incidence*. Despite this 'level playing field' at the outset, the processes by which differential outcomes in CF are generated are unclear. Elucidating these mechanisms is important to inform policies, both to improve care in CF, and to reduce inequalities in health more broadly.

Key Features of Cystic Fibrosis

CF is an inherited, chronic, progressive condition occurring in around 1 in 2500 live births in the UK, and affecting over 9000 individuals, with around 300 new diagnoses annually (Dodge et al. 2007; CF Trust 2013). CF is the commonest serious inherited disease among white populations, and is caused by mutations in the CF transmembrane conductance regulator (CFTR) gene, resulting in thick secretions that impair various organs, particularly the respiratory and digestive systems. It is an autosomal recessive condition; inheritance requires receiving two copies of the defective CFTR gene, one from each parent (Davies et al. 2007). Most children are diagnosed in the first few months of life, and subsequently require intensive support from family and health care services. Most patients die prematurely from their disease through respiratory failure, but with increasing survival into adulthood, CF is best understood as a complex, multisystem disease.

Survival beyond the first few years of life was rare in the 1940s, but UK children born in the twenty-first century are now estimated to have a median survival of over 50 years of age (Dodge et al. 2007). Survival in CF has increased under the influence of improved treatment and management, improved nutrition and better living conditions (Davies et al. 2007; Schechter 2004), but these improvements do not appear to have been shared equally, since studies in both the US and UK have demonstrated differences in survival by socio-economic status (SES) (Schechter et al. 2001; O'Connor et al. 2003; Britton 1989). The social patterning of survival in CF suggests that social factors – the 'social determinants of health' – are having an important effect on outcomes. Utilising some of the unique characteristics of CF to explore the causes of these differences can offer broader insights.

CF is thus an interesting case conceptually for the study of pathways to inequalities in health: as a disease of autosomal recessive inheritance where carriers are unaffected, there is no social bias in incidence (Fig. 5.1), but there is potential for a social gradient in health care use, disease outcome, and social consequences to develop. CF thus opens up opportunities for inequalities research, because it offers both homogeneity, in terms of the population affected by the disease at the outset, and yet great variation in outcomes that can be explored. These two characteristics make for a promising "tracer condition" to improve our understanding of pathways to differential outcomes.

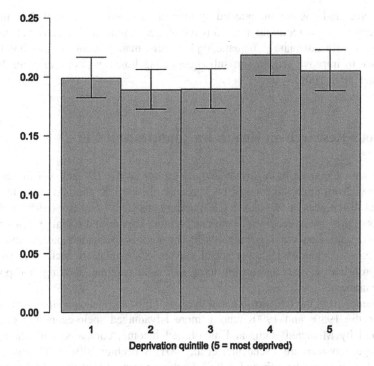

Fig. 5.1 Distribution of incident cases of CF in the UK by deprivation quintile 1996–2010. *Error bars represent 95 % binomial CIs (n = 2066)* (Source: Adapted from Taylor-Robinson et al. 2013b)

Clinical Management of CF

Describing the management of CF in any depth is beyond the scope of this chapter, but for a succinct review see Davies and colleagues (2007). In brief, the key treatment outcomes considered in the analysis relate to respiratory and nutritional therapies:

- Treatment of respiratory infections with antibiotics is a central pillar of CF therapy including for prophylaxis; eradication of infections; long-term treatment of chronic infection, and treatment of acute exacerbations. The aim is to prevent initial bacterial infection in children, and promptly treat acute infections using antibiotics. Acute chest infections (exacerbations) are treated with oral, nebulised, and/or IV antibiotics.
- DNase is an inhaled mucolytic that breaks down the thick sputum in the lungs. This was first commercially available in 1992, and was the first treatment to demonstrate an improvement in lung function in CF (Fuchs et al. 1994).
- The main aims of nutritional support in CF are to achieve optimal nutritional status, and allow normal growth and development throughout childhood. Pancreatic enzyme insufficiency leads to malabsorption of fats, diarrhoea, and failure

to thrive, and this is compounded by lung disease and infection, which further increases calorie requirements. Thus recommendations are for early nutritional support with adequate pancreatic replacement management, as this has been shown to improve growth and subsequent lung function (Konstan et al. 2003; Munck et al. 2009).

Previous Research on Health Inequalities and CF

People with CF from more disadvantaged groups in the UK and US die earlier than those from more advantaged backgrounds. In the UK, the first study to look at social differences in survival in CF found a consistent trend from 1959 to 1986 towards higher age at death in CF patients in more advantaged social groups on the basis of occupational class (Britton 1989). The authors speculated that the observed lower survival chances in lower social classes could relate to lack of access to the appropriate services, poorer nutrition, increased parental smoking, and poorer quality housing.

Evidence from the US corroborated these findings, and indicated higher survival rates in the 1980s and 1990s among more advantaged socio-economic groups, measured by Medicaid status and area-based income, compared with their less advantaged counterparts (Schechter et al. 2001; Schechter 2004; O'Connor et al. 2003). For instance the adjusted risk of death was around four times higher in CF patients with Medicaid cover (used as a surrogate for poverty) compared to those without Medicaid cover (Schechter et al. 2001). Two studies from the US showed differences in lung function on the basis of measures of SES. For instance Schechter et al. also showed significantly lower percent predicted forced expiratory volume in one second (%FEV$_1$) at age 5 in the Medicaid patients (9.2 percentage points, 95 % CI 7.1–11.4), and this gap increased slightly in an age dependent manner up to age 20. O'Connor et al. extended the work of Schechter's team by demonstrating a social gradient in the relationship between area-based income in the US, and mortality rates, lung function and weight (O'Connor et al. 2003). The authors point out the limitations of the ecological (area-based) measure of SES used in their analysis, and suggest that the associations observed may be due to poor adherence to medications, or local environmental conditions.

In many chronic illnesses, differences in access to specialist health care by SES are evident. These differences often contribute to the exacerbation of health inequalities, since a bias towards more advantaged groups is widespread across health care (Stirbu et al. 2011). This could be particularly important in the context of inequalities in outcomes for a disease like CF, where treatment advances have had such a profound effect on survival. The studies exploring access to services and treatments in CF have been predominantly from the US, and have demonstrated a mixed picture, depending on the type of treatment under consideration, and the exact measure of SES used (O'Connor et al. 2003; Schechter et al. 2009, 2011). For instance, one study showed greater access to intravenous (IV) antibiotics for older children, on the basis of area-based income, but also showed no difference in access to DNase, another important treatment in CF, using Medicaid status as a measure of SES (Schechter et al. 2009). Overall the US studies have played down the role of health service factors in the generation of health disparities in CF. However, it is debatable how much of this evidence can be generalized to other health care settings, especially to the UK context, where access to health services is free at the point of use.

Using the Diderichsen Model to Study Inequalities in CF Outcomes in the UK

To gain a better understanding of when and how inequalities in outcomes develop in cystic fibrosis in a UK context, the studies summarised in the subsequent sections of this chapter explored the effect of deprivation on growth, nutrition, lung function, risk of *Pseudomonas aeruginosa* colonisation, and the use of major cystic fibrosis treatment modalities in a UK-wide population cohort, in the context of a the British NHS, a universal healthcare system, free at the point of use (Taylor-Robinson 2013; Taylor-Robinson et al. 2013a, b).

The studies involved longitudinal analyses of individual level patient data from the UK CF Registry, which is supported and co-ordinated by the UK CF Trust (2013; Adler et al. 2008), and records information about the health and treatment of patients with CF from diagnosis onwards. The Registry is estimated to include nearly all people with CF in the UK population (Mehta et al. 2004) and is therefore ideally suited to the study of outcomes and treatments across the whole socio-economic spectrum in the UK society. The studies use postcodes to link individuals to small area deprivation measures in the UK as a measure of socio-economic status (SES), since individual level measures of patient SES, such as parental education level, were not available. The indices of multiple deprivation combine economic, social and housing indicators measured at the census into a fine grained composite deprivation score for small areas in the UK constituent countries (ONS 2011).

The analyses were informed by the Diderichsen model of pathways to health inequalities (Diderichsen et al. 2001). This model captures key concepts in our contemporary understanding of how health inequalities are generated, and was used as the conceptual basis for the work of the WHO Commission for Social Determinants of Health (CSDH 2008). The framework conceptualises the generation of health inequalities occurring through four main pathways over the life course (Fig. 5.2): through social stratification itself, which is the process by which people are sorted into different social positions (for example by social inequalities in the education system); because social stratification leads to differential exposure to risk factors (for example children living in poverty are more likely to be exposed to second-hand smoke in the home); differential vulnerability at the same level of exposure (for example due to clustering of cardiovascular risk factors, smoking is more harmful

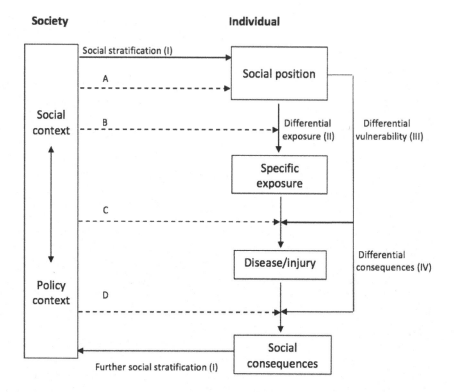

Policy entry points:
A=modifying effect of social context and policy on social stratification;
B=policies affecting differential exposure;
C=policies affecting differential vulnerability;
D=policies affecting differential social consequences of disease.

Fig. 5.2 A conceptual model for studying the effect of social position and social context on health (Adapted from Diderichsen et al. 2001)

to health in the presence of high blood pressure (Capewell and Graham 2010)); and differential consequences of ill health (for example less advantaged groups who experience cardiovascular events are more likely to become unemployed than individuals in more advantaged positions (Holland et al. 2009)).

A key feature of the Diderichsen model is that it incorporates both social causation and social selection mechanisms within a common framework, across the life course. Importantly, the model also explicitly links the broader social environment to the causal pathway at the individual level and makes it clear that the social determinants of health are policy sensitive (Taylor-Robinson 2013).

Using the Diderichsen model, the studies outlined here explored how the clinical consequences of CF vary in the UK on the basis of SES across the life course, and how exposure to health damaging risk factors such as acquisition of important lung infections, and use of major CF treatment modalities vary over time.

A neglected area of study has been the effect of SES on social outcomes in CF, such as employment status. Understanding the *social consequences* of ill health is a key step in elucidating the pathways to health inequalities, since any adverse social outcomes that occur as a result of ill health can feedback and further damage health status. For example, ill health might lead to job loss, which can then have further adverse effects on health status, mediated by a range of physical and psycho-social mechanisms. Furthermore, there is evidence from social epidemiological studies to suggest that, in many settings, it is people from more disadvantaged backgrounds who particularly experience adverse health outcomes as a result of ill health – so called differential social consequences in the Diderichsen model (Milton et al. 2006; Holland et al. 2009; Carlsen et al. 2007, 2008).

The Effect of Socioeconomic Status on Clinical Outcomes in Cystic Fibrosis in the UK

In the UK studies, children with CF from more disadvantaged areas were shown to have worse growth and lung function trajectories compared with children from more affluent areas, but these inequalities did not widen with advancing age (Table 5.1). Looking at growth in the UK CF population in more detail, Fig. 5.3 shows clinically important differences for weight, height BMI on the basis of area deprivation. In a longitudinal analysis, adjusting for a range of confounding factors, the difference in weight and height standard deviation (SD) score is about one third between the most and least advantaged quintiles, whereas for BMI the difference is about one sixth of a standard deviation score (z-score). These results show that having CF, and living in the most disadvantaged areas of the UK effectively doubles the nutritional disadvantage experienced by a person with CF. The deprivation gap in weight is greatest in the first few months of life, at the time of diagnosis, and there follows narrowing of the gap up to around age 3 from around -0.54 SD scores (95 % CI -0.73 to -0.34) at birth to -0.28 (95 % CI -0.38 to -0.18) at age 3, but then the gap remains constant into adulthood (Fig. 5.4).

The finding of a social gradient in growth outcomes, evident from around the time of diagnosis, points to important effects of deprivation in utero, and/or in the initial period prior to diagnosis. Both are plausible, but a limitation of studies thus far has been a lack of data on birth-weight, which would complete the picture. The association between low SES and low birth-weight, and length is well established in the general population (Spencer et al. 1999; Marmot et al. 2010; Howe et al. 2011, 2012). The causes for this are likely to be multi-factorial and relate to maternal health, including stress, diet, drug, alcohol and tobacco use during pregnancy (Marmot et al. 2010). The question remains, however, as to how having CF modifies this relationship. Direct comparison of the SES effect on

Table 5.1 Summary of adjusted effects of deprivation on clinical outcomes and use of therapies in the paediatric and adult CF population in the UK

	Age < 18	Age 18–40
Clinical outcomes[a]		
Lung function as measured by percent predicted forced expiratory volume – %FEV$_1$ (%)	−4·12 (−5·01 to −3·19)	−1·6 (−4·41 to 1·25)
Weight-for-age (SD score)	−0·28 (−0·38 to −0·18)	−0·31 (−0·46 to −0·16)
Height-for-age (SD score)	−0·31 (−0·40 to −0·21)	−0·31 (−0·43 to −0·19)
BMI-for-age (SD score)	−0·13 (−0·22 to −0·04)	−0·12 (−0·25 to 0·01)
OR for *P. aeruginosa* colonisation	1·89 (1·34 to 2·66)	1·78 (1·26 to 2·51)
Therapies		
OR for any IV therapy[b]	2·52 (1·92 to 3·17)	1·89 (1·51 to 2·38)
Mean difference IV days per year (%)[b]	15·9 (8·2 to 24)	10·6 (2·5 to 19·2)
OR for supplemental feeding[c]	1·78 (1·42 to 2·2)	2·38 (1·69 to 3·36)
OR for DNase therapy[b]	0·40 (0·21 to 0·72)	0·37 (0·26 to 0·52)
OR for inhaled antibiotics[c]	0·66 (0·47 to 0·93)	0·40 (0·31 to 0·5)

Source: Adapted from Taylor-Robinson et al. (2013a)

All estimates compare the most deprived quintile to the least deprived (reference) quintile. 95 % CI in parenthesis

[a]The outcomes are from separate longitudinal models adjusted for time trends, sex, genotype, screening status and ethnicity

[b]Adjusted for time trends, sex, genotype, screening status, %FEV$_1$ and *P. aeruginosa colonisation status*

[c]Adjusted for time trends, sex, genotype, screening status and BMI SD score

growth in the CF population, and the general population is challenging, due to the lack of studies using comparable SES measures and birth cohorts, and due to the effect of the obesity epidemic in the general population, whereby a relationship between overweight and low SES emerges from around age 4 onwards (Howe et al. 2011, 2012). This is in contrast to CF, where children are consistently underweight compared to the UK reference population (Taylor-Robinson et al. 2013a). Further data on SES gradients in birth-weight in CF would clarify the extent to which the early growth differentials demonstrated are a reflection of the broader SES effects on birth-weight in the general population. The narrowing of inequality in weight SD score in the first 3 years of life is an important finding and suggests that diagnosis and treatment for CF in the NHS may be having a pro-poor, or 'levelling-up' effect on health inequalities. This has policy implications, and supports the universal screening that has been introduced in the UK to allow earlier diagnosis (Taylor-Robinson 2013).

Lung function, as measured by percent predicted forced expiratory volume in one second (%FEV$_1$) is considered one of the most important clinical outcomes in CF, and Fig. 5.5 shows the differences between deprivation quintiles in the UK with respect to key respiratory outcomes. In an adjusted longitudinal analysis (Table 5.1), people from the most deprived areas had significantly worse lung function (−4.12

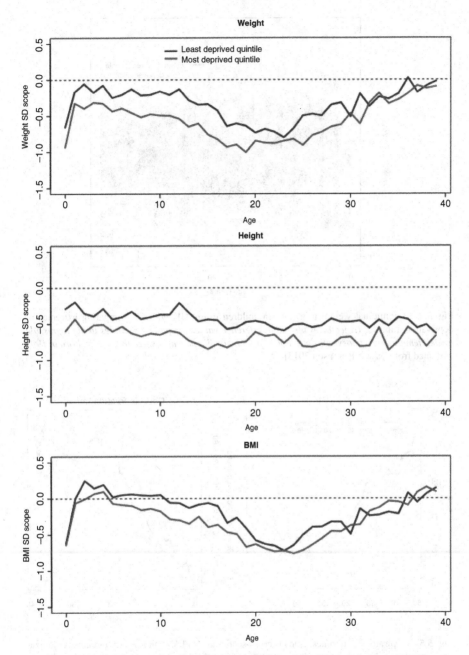

Fig. 5.3 Anthropometric outcomes: mean cross-sectional weight, height, and BMI by age comparing extremes of deprivation quintile (*red* most deprived) (Adapted from Taylor-Robinson et al. 2013a)

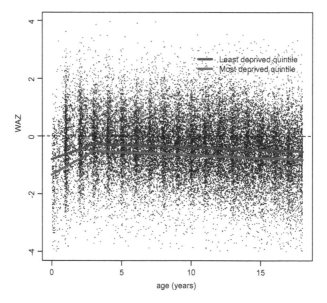

Fig. 5.4 Longitudinal weight trajectory in children in the UK with CF comparing extremes of deprivation quintile. *Trajectories plotted at reference values for other covariates in the regression model: female sex, homozygote delta F508 carrier, not diagnosed by screening, white, born in 1991* (Adapted from Taylor-Robinson 2013)

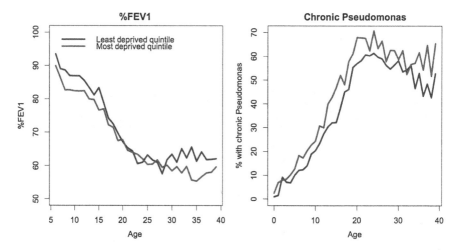

Fig. 5.5 Respiratory outcomes: mean cross-sectional %FEV$_1$ and *P. aeruginosa* colonization prevalence by age comparing extremes of deprivation quintile (Adapted from Taylor-Robinson et al. 2013a)

percentage points, 95 % C1 −5.01 to −3.19), but the deprivation gap in %FEV$_1$ did not increase over the paediatric age range. The prevalence of chronic P. aeruginosa colonisation, the key infection in CF, is also higher in people from the most deprived areas of the UK, from an early age (OR 1.89 in the <18 age group, 95 % CI 1.34 to 2.66) (Table 5.1).

The finding of a social gradient in lung function at age 5 in the UK, when it can be first measured on a routine basis, points to the influence of risk factors earlier in the life course. These are likely to include both environmental and healthcare factors. Schechter and colleagues' found that inequalities in %FEV$_1$ by Medicaid status widened slightly from 5 to 20 years of age (Schechter et al. 2001) in a cross sectional analysis. At round age 5 there was a gap of around 9 % in %FEV1 in the US population, whereas in another study O'Connor and colleagues found a difference of 5.5 % between most and least deprived quintiles (O'Connor et al. 2003). Due to the methodological differences it is not possible to make a direct comparison between UK and US findings in terms of the magnitude of the deprivation gap in lung function (Taylor-Robinson 2013).

In the adult population, growth and P. aeruginosa outcomes were worse in the most deprived adults, but no significant difference in lung function was detected (Table 5.1). The lack of an association between SES and %FEV$_1$ in the adult population is perhaps surprising, given the tendency for social inequalities in health outcomes to increase over time. This may relate to the differences in the use of therapies across social groups described in the next section, or to factors relating to the CF registry, such as left-censoring, selective dropout due to death, and reduced power to detect effects in the adult age range due to the smaller numbers of individuals in the analysis (Taylor-Robinson 2013).

The Effect of Socioeconomic Status on Treatment and Healthcare Use in the UK

Use of IV antibiotic therapy for the treatment of respiratory infections, and clinical exacerbations is a major treatment modality in CF. Longitudinal analysis showed that people in the UK from more deprived areas are about twice as likely to receive IV antibiotics in a particular year, after adjustment for disease severity, on the basis of %FEV$_1$ and P. aeruginosa colonisation status (Odds ratio 2.52, 95 % CI 1.92–3.17 in the <18 age group, and OR 1.89, 95 % CI 1.51–2.38 in the adult age group, comparing most to least deprived quintiles) (Table 5.1, Fig. 5.6). This apparent positive discrimination persists across the age range, from infancy up to 40 years of age. Furthermore if children and adults with CF are recorded as having any IV therapy in a particular year, then people from most deprived areas in the UK, compared to the least, are more likely to have more treatment days (more intensive treatment), after adjusting for disease severity (15.9 % more days in the paediatric age group, 95 % CI 8.2–24, and 10.6 % more days in the adult age group 95 %

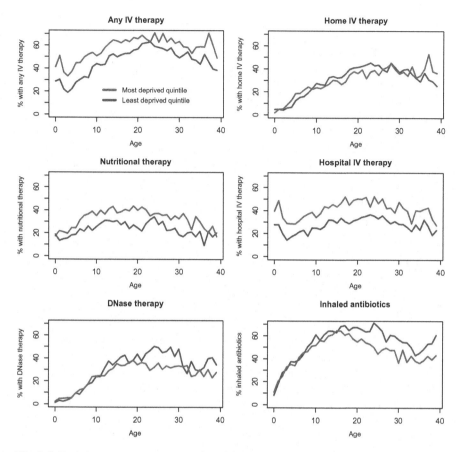

Fig. 5.6 Use of therapies: any IV antibiotic therapy, home IV antibiotic therapy, hospital IV antibiotic therapy, supplemental feeding, DNase, and inhaled antibiotics, by age comparing extremes of deprivation quintile (Source: Adapted from Taylor-Robinson et al. 2013a)

CI 2.5–19.2). Disaggregating the use of any IV antibiotics into use of therapies at home, and in hospital, demonstrated that the positive discrimination in use of any IV therapy was almost entirely due to delivery of these therapies in hospital, as opposed to home-based treatment. Overall, children from more affluent areas were more likely to be treated at home compared to their more disadvantaged counterparts (Fig. 5.6).

The picture is similar for nutritional therapies, with people from more deprived areas of the UK with CF being more likely to be treated with nutritional therapies, after adjustment for nutritional status, measured on the basis of BMI SD score (OR 1.78, 95 % CI 1.42–2.2 in the <18 age group, and OR 2.38, 95 % CI 1.69–3.36 in the adult age group, comparing the most to the least deprived quintiles).

A different pattern is observed when it comes to use of long term inhaled therapies such as DNase and inhaled antibiotics. There was evidence of inequality in the delivery of inhaled therapies to the UK CF population, after adjusting for measures of disease severity (Table 5.1, Fig. 5.6). Furthermore, this association becomes stronger in the adult age range. In children, there was no association between DNase use and deprivation, prior to adjustment for disease severity. However, after adjustment for disease severity, there was an apparent inequality, suggesting that DNase may not be delivered equitably in children. This analysis was clear in the adult population in both the unadjusted and adjusted associations, with adults from more affluent areas being more likely to report using DNase or inhaled antibiotics in the preceding year.

With regard to the major treatments for CF, the UK studies provide evidence of more intensive treatment being delivered to both children and adults with CF, for two major pillars of CF care – treatment with IV therapies, and nutritional therapies – after adjusting for measures of disease severity. These findings provide evidence of a so-called 'pro-poor' bias (Ravallion 2001). Aside from the possibility of residual confounding by severity, one explanation for these findings is that clinicians in the UK are actively taking steps to address, and overcome the perceived excess disadvantage faced by people living in more deprived areas. This may be particularly the case with regard to paediatric care which may be delivered more intensively, and in a hospital setting, to children with CF who are perceived to be living in more disorganised home circumstances, where there may be additional barriers to ensuring that they receive the care and treatments needed (Gupta et al. 2009). More intensive delivery of treatment to more disadvantaged children may further play a role in the reduction in weight inequality over the first few years of life, and the relatively stable inequalities gap demonstrated in the UK studies, as opposed to a finding of increasing inequality.

Longitudinal Employment Status in People with CF

People with chronic illnesses face numerous barriers to entering the labour market, and CF provides a case in point. Factors related to disease severity, such as reduced lung function may restrict employment choices for adults with CF, and the treatment burden further compounds this; adults with CF are generally expected to perform physiotherapy regularly and there are the added demands of taking large numbers of therapies, including frequent visits to hospital (Sawicki et al. 2009).

The analysis of the UK Registry shows that at any one time, about 50 % of the UK CF population was recorded as being in full or part-time employment for all ages, but patterns differed by age, sex, and deprivation status. In a longitudinal analysis, all other things being equal, people from more disadvantaged areas in the UK were less likely to be in employment, and furthermore, social deprivation was found to modify the effect of disease severity in CF: poor lung function, as measured by lower lung function ($\%FEV_1$), is more harmful to employment chances for people living in the most disadvantaged circumstances compared to the least (Fig. 5.7, Table 5.2). A fall in lung function in people with CF has more of an effect on employment

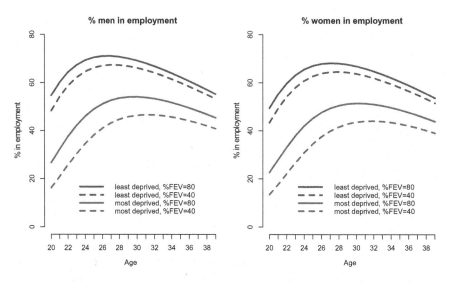

Fig. 5.7 Longitudinal employment trajectory versus age, demonstrating the interaction between deprivation and %FEV₁. *The lines show the final modelled longitudinal contrasting the adjusted effects of deprivation, and %FEV₁. Low %FEV₁is more damaging to employment chances in people living in the most disadvantaged areas. Other covariates in the final model are fixed* (Adapted from Taylor-Robinson et al. 2013b)

Table 5.2 Percentage of people with CF in employment at age 30

	Employment (%)	Employment (%)
	Men	Women
No health or social disadvantage (good lung function and high SES)	69·2	66·8
Health disadvantage only (poor lung function and high SES)	66·1	63·7
Social disadvantage only (good lung function and low SES)	54·1	51·4
Double disadvantage (poor lung function and low SES)	46·4	43·6

Adapted from Taylor-Robinson (2013)
%FEV₁ fixed at 80 percentage points for good lung function, and 40 percentage points for poor lung function
High SES fixed at least deprived quintile, and low SES fixed at most deprived quintile

chances in disadvantaged populations – at the age of 30, a contrast of 40 percentage points in lung function corresponds to a decline in employment prevalence from 69.2 to 66.1 % (3.1 percentage points difference) for men in least deprived quintile, compared to a change from 54.1 to 46.4 % (7.7 percentage points difference) in the most deprived quintile (Table 5.2).

The social consequences of having a chronic disease such as CF are important, and understudied. Although social conditions do not influence the risk of having CF, there are significant differences in outcomes such as growth and lung function, and ultimately survival, in people with CF in the UK and US (Taylor-Robinson et al. 2013a; Schechter et al. 2001; Barr and Fogarty 2011). The analysis of UK data presented here suggests that people with the double burden of chronic illness and low SES are more likely to be excluded from the labour market. This in turn is likely to lead to an increased risk of poverty, social exclusion, and further adverse effects on health. In this way, the *differential social consequences of illness* in the context of CF, represents an important pathway for the amplification of health inequalities over the life course (Taylor-Robinson et al. 2013b).

Social Inequalities, Even for Genetic Diseases

The analyses of the UK CF registry presented here demonstrate that people from more disadvantaged areas in the UK have worse health and social outcomes than their more affluent counterparts. They are more likely to have poor growth, poorer lung function, and to acquire *P. aeruginosa*, and are less likely to be in employment. In contrast, the use of major therapies in the UK CF population shows a so called 'pro-poor' bias, with people living in the most deprived areas of the UK around twice as likely to be treated with IV antibiotics and nutritional therapies, after adjusting for disease severity. However, there was evidence of inequalities in the use of home IV therapies, DNase, and inhaled antibiotics. With regard to employment outcomes the analyses demonstrate that deprivation modifies the effect of disease severity in CF: poor lung function is more harmful to employment chances for people living in the most disadvantaged circumstances compared to the least.

CF is the archetypal classically inherited genetic disease, caused by a single gene defect that is both a necessary and sufficient cause of a chronic illness. CF was one of the first diseases for which the precise genetic mechanism was elucidated, with the sequencing of the CFTR gene, and yet knowledge of the genetic mutation does not predict clinical outcome (Kerem et al. 1990; Schechter 2004). Despite the genetic origin of CF, the evidence presented here shows that outcomes in CF are socially patterned, demonstrating that social factors are leading to profound differences in the course of the illness, which cannot be explained by genetic differences.

Inequalities from the Start

The finding that inequalities start early in the life course for people with CF and then track through until later life, even for a genetic disease like CF, supports the growing evidence around the early origins of health inequalities. The convergence between the inequalities literature, and the current direction of CF research is also striking, whereby both disciplines are suggesting that the early years are critical. In their recent piece on early lung disease, for instance, Grasemann and Ratjen state (Greasemann and Ratjen 2013):

> The infant and preschool age could represent a unique period of opportunity to postpone or even prevent the onset of cystic fibrosis lung disease.

Compare this to possibly the key recommendation of the UK Marmot review (Marmot et al. 2010):

> Action to reduce health inequalities must start before birth and be followed through the life of the child. Only then can the close links between early disadvantage and poor outcomes throughout life be broken.

The findings presented here support the growing consensus that early disadvantage tracks forward, to influence adult health in later life, and that children who start behind tend to stay behind (Marmot et al. 2010; Kuh et al. 2004; Galobardes et al. 2008). This has important implications for public health policy, and suggests that children may have optimum or sub-optimum trajectories on the basis of early life experiences. As Fig. 5.8 below illustrates, these early life trajectories can determine the point at which an individual becomes symptomatic for a particular adult chronic disease. Interventions to targeted in the early years may delay the onset of limiting illness in later life.

The Y-axis in Fig. 5.8 represents some general phenomena relating to health development. For instance, this model has been applied to the development of lung health (Kuh et al. 2004), mental health capacity (Kirkwood et al. 2008), and features in a recent Lancet paper in a very similar form with 'behavioural competence' on the Y-axis (Walker et al. 2011).

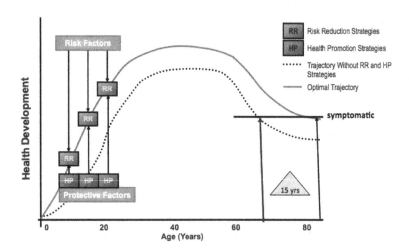

Fig. 5.8 How risk reduction and health promotion strategies influence health development (Adapted from Halfon et al. 2000)

Health Services and Heath Inequalities in CF

The findings presented here have demonstrated variations in the recorded use of treatments by SES for people with CF in the UK NHS. What do these findings tell us more broadly about the role of health services and their role in mitigating or potentiating health inequalities?

An important starting point is to understand what equity in healthcare might look like? Restating Margaret Whitehead's definition, equity in healthcare can be seen as being multifaceted and incorporating ideas about: *fair arrangements that allow equal geographic, economic and cultural access to available services for all in equal need of care.* The end goal of equity in *health care* would be to closely match services to the level of need. This may very well result in large differences in access and use of services between different socioeconomic groups, favouring the more disadvantaged groups in greatest need (Whitehead and Dahlgren 2007).

Need, in the context of the definition above, can be taken to relate not just to disease severity, but also to disadvantage. On this basis one can argue that equity is being achieved for certain aspects of CF care in the NHS, since the data suggests that clinicians are responding to both disease severity, and level of disadvantage when making treatment decisions.

The Commission on Social Determinants of Health highlights that inequitable delivery of health care is an important factor in the generation of health inequalities (CSDH 2008). Whilst health services are generally not the cause of health inequalities (Marmot et al. 2010), they can play an important role in the amplification and perpetuation of disadvantage in a number of ways, for example through the so-called 'inverse care law' (Hart 1971) or the 'medical poverty trap' in health care systems that are not free at the point of access (Whitehead et al. 2001). The famous inverse care law, described by the British GP Tudor Hart (Hart 1971) states:

> The availability of good medical care tends to vary inversely with the need for it in the population served. This inverse care law operates more completely where medical care is exposed to market forces, and less so where such exposure is reduced.

This describes the situation whereby those who most need high quality health care, end up receiving less and/or lower quality care. For this reason, striving for equity in health service delivery, as defined by equal use for equal need (Whitehead and Dahlgren 2007), is a central principle for health care systems (Whitehead 1990), including in the NHS.

In the UK, the Darzi report noted the relationship between low SES and poor health and suggested that the NHS has a pivotal role in providing excellent services as "a matter of fairness" (Darzi 2008). The controversial new Health and Social Care Act further enshrines in legislation explicit duties on the Secretary of State, NHS Commissioning Board and clinical commissioning groups (CCGs) to have regard to the need to *reduce inequalities in access to, and to the outcomes of healthcare* (DH 2012). Many dissenting voices have suggested the legislation is likely to have significant adverse effects on health inequalities (FPH 2010; Pollock et al. 2012a, b; Whitehead et al. 2010). While this may well be the case, the wording of the legislation could serve as a lever to hold those responsible for health services to account in terms of taking action to reduce inequalities in outcomes. In these troubled times for the NHS in the UK, the findings presented here provide some evidence that the system of care in CF can take into account the extra needs of disadvantaged children and their families in the UK to deliver care that may be effective in reducing, or at least limiting an increase in health inequalities.

The analysis also sheds some light on potential differences between the delivery of chronic care for children versus that delivered to adults, by demonstrating an increasing propensity to inequality in delivery of both inhaled CF treatments in the adult population, as compared to the paediatric age group. This corroborates the broader literature, in terms of access to and use of care in chronic diseases, which suggests a different picture in adults and children: In adults, a systematic review of universal health care systems by Hanratty et al. suggested a decline in need adjusted use with increasing deprivation, especially in use of specialist hospital services, but reasonably equitable access to primary health care (Hanratty et al. 2007). A more recent European study found large inequalities in the utilisation of specialist care for chronic diseases, which were not compensated by utilisation of GP services (Stirbu et al. 2011). The analysis of CF Registry data from the UK demonstrated a mixed picture for adults, with marked pro-poor bias for IV and nutritional therapies, but inequality in the use of inhaled therapies.

This contrasts with analyses of children's use of health services in the UK, where the studies have tended to show increased use with lower SES, and arguably equitable delivery of care in the studies that have adjusted for need, notwithstanding the difficulties of undertaking precise adjustment. Cooper et al. found no evidence that children and young people's use of health services varied according to their SES, in an analysis that adjusted for need on the basis of self-reported health status, a rather crude measure, in an analysis of the British General Household survey (Cooper et al. 1998). Saxena et al. demonstrated increased use of primary care for disorders such as infections, asthma, and injuries and poisonings in children with lower SES (Saxena et al. 1999). In a further study by the same author, children's use of primary and secondary health services reflected health status rather than SES, and on this basis the authors suggest that equity of access has been partly achieved (Saxena et al. 2002). A more recent study in the UK demonstrated a clear association between adverse socioeconomic position at the time of birth and increased hospital inpatient admissions, days, and costs during the first 10 years of life (Petrou and Kupek 2005). A further study of children in Nordic countries demonstrated equitable access to primary care, but inequality in use of specialist hospital services after careful adjustment for health status on the basis of questionnaire data (Halldorsson et al. 2002).

It remains unclear whether the increasing inequality observed in use of inhaled treatments in CF in adults reflects general differences between paediatric and adult care for chronic disease, or is specific to differences in the CF model of care, perhaps explained by the potential for paediatricians to act in a more paternalistic manner towards the children in their care, in contrast to the relationship between an adult patient and the CF care team, where adult patients can 'vote with their feet'. Further studies should focus on identifying aspects of CF care in children, and adulthood that may be important in reducing health inequalities.

What Are the Implications for Policy and Clinicians?

For individual clinicians, social deprivation needs to be considered as a major risk factor for poor outcomes in CF, and appropriate responses to remediate against the adverse effects of deprivation should be developed. An important first step is to acknowledge and measure the problem. Without on-going data collection to monitor health inequalities, there can be no policy response.

There are a number of steps that could be taken to influence differential exposures. One obvious target for action is to protect newly diagnosed children from environmental tobacco smoke exposure (ETS), since this may be the single most important explanatory factor for SES-related inequalities in this disease (Taylor-Robinson and Schechter 2011). Early identification of family members who smoke, collection of that data in the registry, and appropriate counselling and referral to smoking cessation services would be an effective intervention for all patients regardless of social position.

The UK analysis presented in this chapter also suggests differential exposure to *P. aeruginosa* acquisition, and this requires further investigation. One concern is that this may relate to hospital-acquired acquisition of *P. aeruginosa*, from other patients with CF, as a result of more time spent in hospital. An appropriate policy response might be to ensure that mechanisms are put in place to facilitate equitable delivery of treatments at home, wherever possible. Home care has been shown to be as effective as hospital treatment for some patients (van Aalderen et al. 1995), but not others (Bosworth and Nielson 1997; Thornton et al. 2005). It is also less expensive and may be associated with improvement in quality of life (van Aalderen et al. 1995). Access to appropriate home care may also mean that children are less likely to miss school, which is important in terms of reducing the differential consequences of ill health.

There are some further steps that individual clinicians and teams could take to reduce children's exposure to poverty, and its consequences. Whilst beyond the scope of full discussion here, an increased focus on a whole family approach to the care of the child with CF, with appropriate involvement of the full range of social services support available to children and families living in disadvantaged circumstances, may help to mitigate some of the effects of social deprivation. This would include supporting parents to access all the benefits and services that they are entitled to, and working to reduce any perceived stigma associated with using these services. Support with the additional costs of childcare, travel to clinic appointments, and any additional medical expenditure would also help reduce the financial burden on the most disadvantaged families. This should be coupled with support to develop patient and family disease self-management skills (Smith and Goldman 2010; Goldman and Smith 2002).

Social workers, and other members of the multidisciplinary CF team have an important role in helping people with CF navigate the welfare system, so that they are clear about the benefits that they are entitled to, and the support available to help people with chronic illness in the workplace. This is particularly important at the moment, in the context of the widespread changes to the welfare and benefits system in the UK, with the drive to reduce the number of people claiming Disability Living Allowance. A recent study by Nash et al. demonstrated that the majority of adult patients with CF claim some benefits, and the majority of these were concerned about the planned reforms (Nash et al. 2011). Furthermore, the concerns of the CF community regarding the changes to the welfare system were outlined in a submission by the CF Trust to the Department of Work and Pensions (2011). Further efforts are required to identify effective workplace, rehabilitation, and other interventions to reduce the employment disadvantage experienced by people with CF, particularly for those from more disadvantaged areas.

A key question for practicing physicians raised by our studies is what role health care delivery plays in mitigating or potentiating health inequalities in CF. In the UK, we have demonstrated a mixed picture, and action is required to understand the inequalities in access to inhaled therapies uncovered, and to promote the pro-poor delivery of care demonstrated for other treatments, that may be effective in limiting increases in outcome inequality over time. The potential utility of systematically targeting more intensive therapy at children living in disadvantaged circumstances should be investigated further (Gupta et al. 2009). The adoption of system-based methods to optimize consistency in the use of best care practices might help further minimize variations in prescribed care (Schechter et al. 2009). Furthermore, the early appearance of inequalities, and the potential for decreasing inequality in weight in the first few years of life, focusses policies on the early years, and provides support for new-born screening programmes in CF.

Ultimately, however, while individually focussed interventions may be of some limited success, the long term solution to health inequalities in people with CF and in the general population is likely to be one that takes broader action to address the "social determinants of health" (CSDH 2008). These are the "conditions in which we are born, grow up, work and live", and include income and income distribution, education, employment and working conditions, housing, food insecurity, race/ethnicity, and gender roles. These factors provide a particularly important context for a family dealing with the stresses of caring for a child with a complex chronic illness like CF over a lifetime. The evidence is clear, unfortunately, that we have made little progress over the last few decades in reducing health inequalities (Marmot et al. 2010). However, the analysis presented in this chapter provides further evidence that the early years represent the key period for targeting interventions to reduce inequalities. An important place to start would be to renew efforts in the UK to reduce children's exposure to poverty, by for instance (Marmot et al. 2010):

• maximising household incomes, by helping parents into employment;
• providing affordable housing;

- providing affordable, high quality child care;
- providing affordable public transport;
- helping families manage debt;
- providing better social security support for families caring for children with chronic illness.

With reference to Fig. 5.8 above, policy makers should also act to reduce any inequitable distribution of health damaging and health promoting exposures over the course of children's lives. Reducing the consequences of poverty by focussing on child development in the early years is a good place to start. Actions could involve (Marmot et al. 2010; Field 2010):

- protecting investment in the early years in the face of budget cuts in the UK;
- shifting expenditure towards the early years wherever possible;
- providing high quality and consistent support and services for parents during pregnancy;
- providing high quality universal services in childhood;
- supporting families to achieve progressive improvements in early child development, by providing good quality early years education and childcare;
- providing support so that all children can access a healthy diet in the early years;
- providing high quality home visiting services;
- focussing on narrowing the educational attainment gap at all stages.

As health deteriorates, the ability of people to remain in education and employment declines. Being out of work increases the risk of poverty and social exclusion, and is likely to further damage the health of the most disadvantaged. Actions to address differential social consequences could include (Holland et al. 2011):

- supporting people with chronic illness to find appropriate employment, with a focus on active labour market policies;
- providing better in-work social security support for people with chronic illness.

Conclusions

CF is the commonest serious inherited disease among Caucasian populations. Intensive support from family and health care services is needed from the time of diagnosis onwards, and most patients die prematurely from respiratory failure. There have been astounding improvements in survival over successive birth cohorts in CF, such that it is estimated that British children born in the twenty-first century will have a median survival of over 50 years of age (Dodge et al. 2007). However, there remains a great deal of variation in disease progression and survival in CF, much of which is related to social and environmental rather than genetic determinants (Schechter 2004). Most pointedly, it has been known for over 20 years (Britton 1989) that people with CF from socio-economically disadvantaged backgrounds die younger than those in more advantaged positions.

CF offers a valuable case for understanding how health inequalities develop. It is an autosomal recessive disease with an asymptomatic (and, until recently, undetectable) carrier state, so unlike many other diseases, SES does not influence who gets CF. SES-related outcome inequalities develop due to the different patterns of exposure to harmful and protective or therapeutic influences over the course of people's lives. Studies from the US and UK show that significant inequalities in key intermediate CF outcomes such as growth and lung function begin early in childhood (Taylor-Robinson et al. 2013a; Schechter et al. 2001; O'Connor et al. 2003) and then persist over time. The early appearance and persistence of inequalities supports the need for interventions that are targeted at the early (and perhaps prenatal) years.

References

Adler, A. I., Shine, B. S., Chamnan, P., Haworth, C. S., & Bilton, D. (2008). Genetic determinants and epidemiology of cystic fibrosis-related diabetes: Results from a British cohort of children and adults. *Diabetes Care, 31*(9), 1789–1794. doi: dc08-0466 [pii] 10.2337/dc08-0466.

Barr, H. L. S. A., & Fogarty, A. W. (2011). The association between socioeconomic status and gender with median age at death from cystic fibrosis in England and Wales: 1959 to 2008. *British Medical Journal, 343*, d4662.

Barr, B., Taylor-Robinson, D., & Whitehead, M. (2012). Impact on health inequalities of rising prosperity in England 1998–2007, and implications for performance incentives: Longitudinal ecological study. *British Medical Journal, 345*, e7831. doi:10.1136/bmj.e7831.

Bosworth, D. G., & Nielson, D. W. (1997). Effectiveness of home versus hospital care in the routine treatment of cystic fibrosis. *Pediatric Pulmonology, 24*(1), 42–47.

Britton, J. R. (1989). Effects of social class, sex, and region of residence on age at death from cystic fibrosis. *British Medical Journal, 298*(6672), 483–487.

Capewell, S., & Graham, H. (2010). Will cardiovascular disease prevention widen health inequalities? *PLoS Medicine, 7*(8), e1000320. doi:10.1371/journal.pmed.1000320.

Carlsen, K., Dalton, S. O., Frederiksen, K., Diderichsen, F., & Johansen, C. (2007). Are cancer survivors at an increased risk for divorce? A Danish cohort study. *European Journal of Cancer, 43*(14), 2093–2099.

Carlsen, K., Dalton, S. O., Diderichsen, F., Johansen, C., & Danish Cohort, S. (2008). Risk for unemployment of cancer survivors: A Danish cohort study. *European Journal of Cancer, 44*(13), 1866–1874. doi:10.1016/j.ejca.2008.05.020.

CF Trust. (2013). *CF registry – annual data reports.* http://www.cysticfibrosis.org.uk/about-cf/publications/cf-registry-reports.aspx. Accessed 25 Apr 2013.

Cooper, H., Smaje, C., & Arber, S. (1998). Use of health services by children and young people according to ethnicity and social class: Secondary analysis of a national survey. *British Medical Journal, 317*(7165), 1047–1051.

CSDH. (2008). *Closing the gap in a generation: Health equity through action on the social determinants of health.* Final report of the commission on social determinants of health. http://whqlibdoc.who.int/publications/2008/9789241563703_eng.pdf. Accessed 29 Aug 2008.

Darzi, A. R. (2008). *High quality care for all: NHS next stage review final report*. London: Department of Health.

Davies, J. C., Alton, E., & Bush, A. (2007). Clinical review: Cystic fibrosis. *British Medical Journal, 335*(7632), 1255.

Department of Work and Pensions. (2011). *Disability living allowance reform – submission by the Cystic Fibrosis Trust*. http://www.dwp.gov.uk/docs/dla-reform-cystic-fibrosis-trust.doc. Accessed 25 Apr 2013.

DH. (2012). *Reducing health inequalities – The health and social care act 2012*. http://www.gov.uk/government/uploads/system/uploads/attachment_data/file/138267/C2.-Factsheet-Tackling-inequalities-in-healthcare-270412.pdf. Accessed 12 Apr 2013.

Diderichsen, F., Evans, T., & Whitehead, M. (2001). The social origins of disparities in health. In T. Evans, M. Whitehead, F. Diderichsen, A. Bhuiya, & M. Wirth (Eds.), *Challenging inequities in health* (pp. 12–23). New York: Oxford University Press.

Dodge, J. A., Lewis, P. A., Stanton, M., & Wilsher, J. (2007). Cystic fibrosis mortality and survival in the UK: 1947–2003. *European Respiratory Journal, 29*(3), 522–526.

Field, F. (2010). *The foundation years: Preventing poor children becoming poor adults*. London: The Stationery Office/Tso.

FPH. (2010). *FPH calls on government to withdraw health and social care bill 'in best interests of everyone's health'*. http://www.fph.org.uk/fph_calls_on_government_to_withdraw_health_and_social_care_bill_\T1\textquoteleftin_best_interests_of_everyone\T1\textquoterights_health\T1\textquoteright. Accessed 12 Mar 2013.

Fuchs, H. J., Borowitz, D. S., Christiansen, D. H., Morris, E. M., Nash, M. L., Ramsey, B. W., Rosenstein, B. J., Smith, A. L., & Wohl, M. E. (1994). Effect of aerosolized recombinant human DNase on exacerbations of respiratory symptoms and on pulmonary function in patients with cystic fibrosis. The Pulmozyme Study Group. *New England Journal of Medicine, 331*(10), 637–642. doi:10.1056/NEJM199409083311003.

Galobardes, B., Lynch, J. W., & Smith, G. D. (2008). Is the association between childhood socioeconomic circumstances and cause-specific mortality established? Update of a systematic review. *Journal of Epidemiology and Community Health, 62*(5), 387–390. doi:10.1136/jech.2007.065508.

Goldman, D. P., & Smith, J. P. (2002). Can patient self-management help explain the SES health gradient? *Proceedings of the National Academy of Sciences of the United States of America, 99*(16), 10929–10934. doi:10.1073/pnas.162086599.

Greasemann, H., & Ratjen, F. (2013). Early lung disease in cystic fibrosis. *The Lancet Respiratory Medicine, 1*(2), 148–157.

Gupta, A., Urquhart, D., & Rosenthal, M. (2009). Marked improvement in cystic fibrosis lung disease and nutrition following change in home environment. *Journal of the Royal Society of Medicine, 102*(Suppl 1), 45–48. doi:10.1258/jrsm.2009.s19010.

Halfon, N., Inkelas, M., & Hochstein, M. (2000). The health development organization: An organizational approach to achieving child health development. *The Milbank Quarterly, 78*(3), 447–497. 341.

Halldorsson, M., Kunst, A. E., Kohler, L., & Mackenbach, J. P. (2002). Socioeconomic differences in children's use of physician services in the Nordic countries. *Journal of Epidemiology and Community Health, 56*(3), 200–204.

Hanratty, B., Zhang, T., & Whitehead, M. (2007). How close have universal health systems come to achieving equity in use of curative services? A systematic review. *International Journal of Health Services, 37*(1), 89–109.

Hart, J. T. (1971). The inverse care law. *Lancet, 1*(7696), 405–412.

Holland, P., Burstrom, B., Moller, I., & Whitehead, M. (2009). Socioeconomic inequalities in the employment impact of ischaemic heart disease: A longitudinal record linkage study in Sweden. *Scandinavian Journal of Public Health, 37*(5), 450–458. doi:10.1177/1403494809106501.

Holland, P., Burstrom, B., Whitehead, M., Diderichsen, F., Dahl, E., Barr, B., Nylen, L., Chen, W. H., Thielen, K., van der Wel, K. A., Clayton, S., & Uppal, S. (2011). How do macro-level contexts and policies affect the employment chances of chronically ill and disabled people? Part I: The impact of recession and deindustrialization. *International Journal of Health Services, 41*(3), 395–413.

Howe, L. D., Tilling, K., Galobardes, B., Smith, G. D., Ness, A. R., & Lawlor, D. A. (2011). Socioeconomic disparities in trajectories of adiposity across childhood. *International Journal of Pediatric Obesity, 6*(2-2), e144–e153. doi:10.3109/17477166.2010.500387.

Howe, L. D., Tilling, K., Galobardes, B., Smith, G. D., Gunnell, D., & Lawlor, D. A. (2012). Socioeconomic differences in childhood growth trajectories: At what age do height inequalities emerge? *Journal of Epidemiology and Community Health, 66*(2), 143–148. doi: jech.2010.113068 [pii] 10.1136/jech.2010.113068.

Kerem, E., Corey, M., Kerem, B. S., Rommens, J., Markiewicz, D., Levison, H., Tsui, L. C., & Durie, P. (1990). The relation between genotype and phenotype in cystic fibrosis–analysis of the most common mutation (delta F508). *New England Journal of Medicine, 323*(22), 1517–1522. doi:10.1056/NEJM199011293232203.

Kirkwood, T., Bond, J., May, C., McKeith, I., & Teh, M. (2008). *Foresight mental capital and wellbeing project. Mental capital through life: Future challenges*. London: Government Office for Science.

Konstan, M. W., Butler, S. M., Wohl, M. E., Stoddard, M., Matousek, R., Wagener, J. S., Johnson, C. A., & Morgan, W. J. (2003). Growth and nutritional indexes in early life predict pulmonary function in cystic fibrosis. *Journal of Pediatrics, 142*(6), 624–630. doi: S0022-3476(03)00059-3 [pii] 10.1067/mpd.2003.152.

Kuh, D., Power, C., Blane, D., & Bartley, M. (2004). A life course approach to chronic disease epidemiology. In D. Kuh, C. Power, D. Blane, & M. Bartley (Eds.), *A life course approach to chronic disease epidemiology* (2nd ed., pp. 371–398). Oxford: Oxford University Press.

Marmot, M. G., Allen, J., Goldblatt, P., Boyce, T., McNeish, D., Grady, M., & Geddes, I. (2010). *Fair society, healthy lives: Strategic review of health inequalities in England post-2010*. London: The Marmot Review.

Mehta, G., Sims, E. J., Culross, F., McCormick, J. D., & Mehta, A. (2004). Potential benefits of the UK cystic fibrosis database. *Journal of the Royal Society of Medicine, 97*(Suppl 44), 60–71.

Milton, B., Holland, P., & Whitehead, M. (2006). The social and economic consequences of childhood-onset Type 1 diabetes mellitus across the lifecourse: A systematic review. *Diabetic Medicine, 23*(8), 821–829.

Munck, A., Duhamel, J. F., Lamireau, T., Le Luyer, B., Le Tallec, C., Bellon, G., Roussey, M., Foucaud, P., Ginies, J. L., Houzel, A., Marguet, C., Guillot, M., David, V., Kapel, N., Dyard, F., & Henniges, F. (2009). Pancreatic enzyme replacement therapy for young cystic fibrosis patients. *Journal of Cystic Fibrosis, 8*(1), 14–18. doi:10.1016/j.jcf.2008.07.003.

Nash, E. F., Kavanagh, D., Williams, S., Bikmalla, S., Gray, A., & Whitehouse, J. L. (2011). Implications of the current UK welfare reforms for adults with cystic fibrosis. *Clinical Medicine, 11*(6), 634.

O'Connor, G. T., Quinton, H. B., Kneeland, T., Kahn, R., Lever, T., Maddock, J., Robichaud, P., Detzer, M., & Swartz, D. R. (2003). Median household income and mortality rate in cystic fibrosis. *Pediatrics, 111*(4 Pt 1), e333–e339.

ONS. (2011). *Indices of deprivation across the UK*. http://www.neighbourhood.statistics.gov.uk/dissemination/Info.do?page=analysisandguidance/analysisarticles/indices-of-deprivation.htm. Accessed 29 July 2011.

Petrou, S., & Kupek, E. (2005). Socioeconomic differences in childhood hospital inpatient service utilisation and costs: Prospective cohort study. *Journal of Epidemiology and Community Health, 59*(7), 591–597. doi:10.1136/jech.2004.025395.

Pollock, A. M., Price, D., & Roderick, P. (2012a). Health and social care bill 2011: A legal basis for charging and providing fewer health services to people in England. *British Medical Journal, 344*, e1729. doi:10.1136/bmj.e1729.

Pollock, A. M., Price, D., Roderick, P., Treuherz, T., McCoy, D., McKee, M., & Reynolds, L. (2012b). How the health and social care bill 2011 would end entitlement to comprehensive health care in England. *Lancet, 379*(9814), 387–389. doi:10.1016/S0140-6736(12)60119-6.

Ravallion, M. (2001). Growth, inequality and poverty: Looking beyond averages. *World Development, 29*(11), 1803–1815.

Sawicki, G. S., Sellers, D. E., & Robinson, W. M. (2009). High treatment burden in adults with cystic fibrosis: Challenges to disease self-management. *Journal of Cystic Fibrosis, 8*(2), 91–96. doi: S1569-1993(08)00145-8 [pii] 10.1016/j.jcf.2008.09.007.

Saxena, S., Majeed, A., & Jones, M. (1999). Socioeconomic differences in childhood consultation rates in general practice in England and Wales: Prospective cohort study. *British Medical Journal, 318*(7184), 642–646.

Saxena, S., Eliahoo, J., & Majeed, A. (2002). Socioeconomic and ethnic group differences in self reported health status and use of health services by children and young people in England: Cross sectional study. *British Medical Journal, 325*(7363), 520.

Schechter, M. S. (2004). Non-genetic influences on CF lung disease: The role of sociodemographic characteristics, environmental exposures and healthcare interventions. *Pediatric Pulmonology, Supplement 26*, 82–85.

Schechter, M. S., Shelton, B. J., Margolis, P. A., & Fitzsimmons, S. C. (2001). The association of socioeconomic status with outcomes in cystic fibrosis patients in the United States. *American Journal of Respiratory and Critical Care Medicine, 163*(6), 1331–1337.

Schechter, M. S., McColley, S. A., Silva, S., Haselkorn, T., Konstan, M. W., & Wagener, J. S. (2009). Association of socioeconomic status with the use of chronic therapies and healthcare utilization in children with cystic fibrosis. *Journal of Pediatrics, 155*(5), 634–639. e631–634. doi: S0022-3476(09)00455-7 [pii] 10.1016/j.jpeds.2009.04.059.

Schechter, M. S., McColley, S. A., Regelmann, W., Millar, S. J., Pasta, D. J., Wagener, J. S., Konstan, M. W., & Morgan, W. J. (2011). Socioeconomic status and the likelihood of antibiotic treatment for signs and symptoms of pulmonary exacerbation in children with cystic fibrosis. *Journal of Pediatrics, 159*(5), 819–824. e811. doi: S0022-3476(11)00483-5 [pii] 10.1016/j.jpeds.2011.05.005.

Smith, J. P., & Goldman, D. (2010). Can patient self-management explain the health gradient? Goldman and Smith (2002) revisited: A response to Maitra. *Social Science and Medicine, 70*(6), 813–815. doi:10.1016/j.socscimed.2009.11.010.

Spencer, N., Bambang, S., Logan, S., & Gill, L. (1999). Socioeconomic status and birth weight: Comparison of an area-based measure with the Registrar General's social class. *Journal of Epidemiology and Community Health, 53*(8), 495–498.

Stirbu, I., Kunst, A. E., Mielck, A., & Mackenbach, J. P. (2011). Inequalities in utilisation of general practitioner and specialist services in 9 European countries. *BMC Health Services Research, 11*, 288. doi: 1472-6963-11-288 [pii] 10.1186/1472-6963-11-288.

Taylor-Robinson, D. C. (2013). *The effect of socio-economic status on outcomes in cystic fibrosis.* Doctoral thesis, University of Liverpool. http://research-archive.liv.ac.uk/13813/. Accessed 4 Apr 2014.

Taylor-Robinson, D., & Schechter, M. S. (2011). Health inequalities and cystic fibrosis. *British Medical Journal, 343*, d4818. doi: 10.1136/bmj.d4818 bmj.d4818 [pii].

Taylor-Robinson, D., Smyth, R. L., Diggle, P., & Whitehead, M. (2013a). The effect of social deprivation on clinical outcomes and the use of treatments in the UK cystic fibrosis population: A longitudinal study. *The Lancet Respiratory Medicine, 1*(2), 121–128.

Taylor-Robinson, D. C., Smyth, R., Diggle, P. J., & Whitehead, M. (2013b). A longitudinal study of the impact of social deprivation and disease severity on employment status in the UK cystic fibrosis population. *PloS One, 8*(8), e73322. doi:10.1371/journal.pone.0073322.

Thornton, J., Elliott, R. A., Tully, M. P., Dodd, M., & Webb, A. K. (2005). Clinical and economic choices in the treatment of respiratory infections in cystic fibrosis: Comparing hospital and home care. *Journal of Cystic Fibrosis, 4*(4), 239–247. doi:10.1016/j.jcf.2005.08.003.

van Aalderen, W. M., Mannes, G. P., Bosma, E. S., Roorda, R. J., & Heymans, H. S. (1995). Home care in cystic fibrosis patients. *European Respiratory Journal, 8*(1), 172–175.

Walker, S. P., Wachs, T. D., Grantham-McGregor, S., Black, M. M., Nelson, C. A., Huff-man, S. L., Baker-Henningham, H., Chang, S. M., Hamadani, J. D., Lozoff, B., Gardner, J. M., Powell, C. A., Rahman, A., & Richter, L. (2011). Inequality in early childhood: Risk and protective factors for early child development. *Lancet, 378*(9799), 1325–1338. doi:10.1016/S0140-6736(11)60555-2.

Whitehead, M. (1990). *The concepts and principles of equity and health.* Copenhagen: WHO, Regional Office for Europe.

Whitehead, M., & Dahlgren, G. (2007). *Concepts and principles for tackling social inequities in health: Levelling up Part 1.* Copenhagen: WHO.

Whitehead, M., Dahlgren, G., & Evans, T. (2001). Equity and health sector reforms: Can low-income countries escape the medical poverty trap? *Lancet, 358*(9284), 833–836. doi:10.1016/S0140-6736(01)05975-X.

Whitehead, M., Hanratty, B., & Popay, J. (2010). NHS reform: Untried remedies for misdiagnosed problems? *Lancet, 376*(9750), 1373–1375. doi:10.1016/S0140-6736(10)61231-7.

Chapter 6
Moving Towards a Better Understanding of Socioeconomic Inequalities in Preventive Health Care Use: A Life Course Perspective

Sarah Missinne

Introduction

Despite the abundance of empirical studies that have targeted a whole range of social groups and (preventive) health services, little remains understood about the underlying mechanisms that drive persistent socioeconomic inequalities in preventive health care use. Recently, cultural health capital and health lifestyles have been discussed theoretically with regard to their roles in preventive health care inequalities. Given substantial analogies, I explore in this chapter how our understanding of cultural health capital and preventive health care inequalities can be advanced by applying the five theoretical principles of the life course perspective as described by Elder and colleagues (2003). The objective is to set out a framework that can be applied to different forms of preventive health care. However, I use the example of mammography screening, as this preventive health habit has been the focus of my empirical research. There are several reasons for this choice. First, breast cancer constitutes a very important public health issue, as it is the most frequently diagnosed form of cancer among European women (Ferlay et al. 2010) and the leading cause of female death from cancer (Ferlay et al. 2013; Jemal 2011). Mammography screening is the only evidence-based method for detecting breast cancer at an early stage (Youlden et al. 2012), and has improved survival rates by 19 to 32 % in several European countries for women in the age range 50 to 69 (Hakama et al. 2008). Socioeconomic inequalities have also been reported with regard to mammography screening (e.g. Duport and Ancelle-Park 2006; Jusot et al. 2011).

S. Missinne (✉)
Department of Sociology, Ghent University, St. Pietersnieuwstraat 33, Ghent 9000, Belgium
e-mail: Sarah.Missinne@UGent.be

© The Author(s) 2015

C. Burton-Jeangros et al. (eds.), *A Life Course Perspective on Health Trajectories and Transitions*, Life Course Research and Social Policies 4,
DOI 10.1007/978-3-319-20484-0_6

The second reason for choosing mammography screening relates to data avail-ability. Information is available about the year in which women commenced regular mammography screening. Unfortunately, information on the timeliness is rare in the field of preventive health care despite the fact that the notion of timing is also a vital aspect of preventive health habits, as is outlined below. This duration data enables us to illustrate the potential of all five life course principles for preventive health care research[1] by means of event history analysis. This statistical technique is commonly used in life course research, as the concept of transition is central to both the theoretical perspective and the statistical modeling of event histories (Wu 2003).

The chapter is structured as follows: first, I outline how preventive health care inequalities have been approached traditionally, before focusing in detail on cultural health capital theory and health lifestyle theory. Each of the five principles of the life course perspective and their potential application and similarities with preventive health care research are elaborated upon separately, although there is unavoidably some overlap. Each time, I refer to previous empirical work to illustrate the empirical application of a particular principle using the example of mammography screening.

Theoretical Models on Preventive Health Care Inequalities

Traditional Approaches to Preventive Health Care Inequalities

To assess socioeconomic inequalities in preventive health care use, the need-adjusted approach based on Andersen's heuristic model of health service use (Andersen et al. 1970; revised form: Andersen 1995) is generally relied upon. Researchers define and adjust for indicators of 'need' and subsequently assess whether socioeconomic inequalities in health care use persist. Inequity arises, for example, if individuals in higher socioeconomic groups are more likely to use, or are using, a greater quantity of health services – after controlling for their level of ill-health – compared with that of lower socioeconomic groups (van Doorslaer et al. 2006).

In addition to the need-adjusted approach of Andersen (1970, 1995), socioeco-nomic differences in preventive health care use have traditionally been explained by theoretical models of health behavior, such as the widely-used health belief model (Becker and Maiman 1975) and the theory of reasoned action (Fishbein and Ajzen 1975). Importantly, these models highlight the role of beliefs (about perceived risks,

---

[1] The other side of the coin is that the effectiveness of mammography screening continues to be a widely-debated prevention strategy (Gotzsche and Nielsen 2009), despite general guidelines by the WHO (2013) and the European Union. Although this renders the discussion somewhat more complex on several points, it does not hinder us in our aim to set up a new framework for preventive health care research.

severity, efficacy of personal action, benefits, and costs) in preventive health care use, and contend that use is not determined by financial means alone, as is often assumed when adopting a need-adjusted approach (Rajaram and Rashidi 1998). However, these agency-oriented paradigms lack an understanding of how beliefs are socially and culturally structured (Blane 2008; Frohlich et al. 2001; Rajaram and Rashidi 1998) and how they are acquired over the course of an individual's life. In twenty-first century medical sociology, there is now a growing awareness that understanding the true social rooting of health and illness requires a shift from the dominant agency-oriented paradigms towards a more neo-structural perspective (Cockerham 2005, 2007).

Cultural (Health) Capital Theory

Recent theoretical developments have aimed to underline the structural dimension of health and health care habits. A central element is the conceptualization of social position. Scholars have argued that in current post-industrial societies, stratification is not driven by social class alone (Clark and Lipset 2001). As a result of better labor conditions, increasing wages, and disposable time, consumption patterns have gained importance (Bogenhold 2001). Therefore, the explicit inclusion of cultural capital in explanatory approaches to social inequality in health and health behavior has been advocated, rather than deducing it from general measurements of socioeconomic status (SES), such as social class and income (Abel 2008; Abel and Frohlich 2012; Shim 2010). Bourdieu (1986) described how inequality could be reproduced by the interplay of three different forms of capital: economic, social, and cultural. He further identified three different forms of cultural capital: objectivized (e.g. books, artefacts, paintings), institutionalized (e.g. education, job title) and the embodied state incorporating mind and body (e.g. values, skills, knowledge).

When applying Bourdieu's (1986) general notion of cultural capital to health and health care research, what is termed cultural health capital can be defined as comprising "all culture-based resources that are available to people for acting in favour of their health. In its incorporated form it comprises health-related values, behavioural norms, knowledge and operational skills" (Abel 2008, p. 2). This form of cultural capital becomes directly relevant to health through the adoption of healthy lifestyles, such as engaging in preventive care (Abel 2008; Abel and Frohlich 2012; Phelan et al. 2004; Shim 2010).

Analogous to life course research, a longer view of an individual's life is taken when elaborating on how cultural health capital develops. It has been argued that the health-relevant knowledge and skills used to lead healthy lives start accumulating in childhood and this proceeds over the life course through repeated contacts with health care providers and lifelong socialization (Abel and Frohlich 2012; Mirowsky and Ross 2003; Shim 2010). Cultural health capital theory highlights that people's behavioral options and preferences are structurally constrained and unequally distributed between social groups (Abel 2008).

Health Lifestyle Theory

In the same theoretical tradition, Cockerham (2005, 2007) developed the 'health lifestyle theory' to underline the structural dimensions of health lifestyles. Starting from Weber's lifestyle concept (Weber [1922] 1978), Cockerham described health lifestyles as "collective patterns of health-related behaviour based on choices from options available to people according to their life chances" (Cockerham 2000, p. 165). Health lifestyles are largely shared by individuals close to one another in a social space, and whose similar opportunities in terms of life chances give rise to a shared general habitus as elaborated by Bourdieu. In *La Distinction* (1984), he outlined how this dialectic interplay between life choices and life chances gives rise to a set of lifestyle dispositions, which make up the habitus of individuals. Members of the same social class are more likely to share the same general habitus, because they internalize the same life chances. Hence, choices of health lifestyles are not uncoordinated, but are largely shared by social class members (Cockerham 2005, 2007) and are likely to be transmitted intergenerationally (Wickrama et al. 1999). Bourdieu's notion of habitus (1984) entails that "health-related behaviour can be seen as a largely routinized feature of everyday life which is guided by a practical or implicit logic" (Williams 1995, p. 583). Therefore, not every use of available resources, including cultural health capital, is as conscious as traditional models of health behavior assume (Abel and Frohlich 2012; Shim 2010).

Cockerham (2007) highlighted that notwithstanding their own complexities, health practices comprise an overall pattern, accordingly the regular take-up of preventive mammography screening can be viewed as an expression of a health lifestyle that started to develop during childhood. There is also empirical support for a general behavioral orientation towards a health lifestyle (Donovan et al. 1993).

Preventive Health Care Inequalities Along the Five Principles of the Life Course Perspective

Principle 1: Life-Span Development

The life course perspective is distinctive for its extended time frame and its focus on evolving dynamics that begin in early childhood (Elder et al. 2003). A key issue that is addressed is the sociogenesis of inequality between people over the life course (Schafer et al. 2011). Early advantage or disadvantage can set in motion a series of cascading socioeconomic and lifestyle events that have consequences across different domains in later life, such as education (Gamoran and Mare 1989) and work (Gangl 2004). More recently, the life course perspective has also been introduced in social epidemiology by Blane (1999), Kuh and colleagues (2003), and Halfon and Hochstein (2002). Studies have already revealed that early or midlife factors, such as childhood socioeconomic conditions and health, have long-term influences on adult health and mortality (Due et al. 2011; Hayward and Gorman 2004), and healthy ageing (Brandt et al. 2011). However, the role of the life course perspective in terms of preventive health care use still needs to be assessed.

Cultural health capital theorists have implicitly adopted the idea of life-span development. Yet, the way in which cultural health capital is acquired and how it evolves over time remain unexplored (Shim 2010). We are in the dark regarding whether and which specific life stages or experiences are crucial in the development of cultural health capital or health lifestyles (Singh-Manoux and Marmot 2005). Pioneering empirical studies on cultural health capital have been conducted (e.g. Dubbin et al. 2013). However, the developmental dimension of cultural health capital has not yet received much attention.

Childhood socioeconomic conditions can shape the development of health-related behaviors (Kuh et al. 2004) when parents transfer skills and knowledge to their children (Abel and Frohlich 2012; Singh-Manoux and Marmot 2005). In addition to setting an example by buying food, (alcoholic) beverages, engaging in sports, taking their children for regular dental check-ups, etc., the beliefs supporting parents' own health behavior are transmitted unintentionally or via explicit teaching efforts (Lau et al. 1990; Tinsley et al. 2002).

The SHARELIFE[2] data enables the initial empirical testing of cultural health capital theory by including several unique measurements (see Missinne et al. 2014 for methodological details). The main question posed here is whether childhood is a decisive period in the development of preventive health behavior. Empirically, it is assessed whether cultural health capital in childhood, as approximated by childhood preventive behavior, predicts the take-up of mammography screening many years later in life. Figure 6.1 indeed shows that women who went to the dentist regularly for preventive check-ups during childhood are more likely, at every age, to take-up regular mammography screenings. The log-rank test confirms that this bivariate association is significant (p<0.001). To what extent is this association attributable to a more prosperous socioeconomic situation in childhood? The multivariate models[3] demonstrate that engaging in preventive health behavior during childhood is associated with an increased hazard of mammography screening of 45 %, regardless of traditional socioeconomic factors of childhood (the ISCO-88 of the main breadwinner's job and the number of books in the household). This early-life advantage only decreases slightly (15.6 % = 0.38–0.45/0.45) when the adulthood socioeconomic position (wealth and education) is additionally taken into account. As suggested by the full-path dependence model (DiPrete and Eirich

[2]The Survey of Health, Ageing and Retirement (SHARE, www.share-project.org) is a multi-disciplinary and cross-national panel database on health, socioeconomic status, and social and family networks. The third wave which provides retrospective life course information, is used (SHARELIFE)

[3]The models all account for cohort and period effects as well as the age-eligibility for the Belgian national screening program.

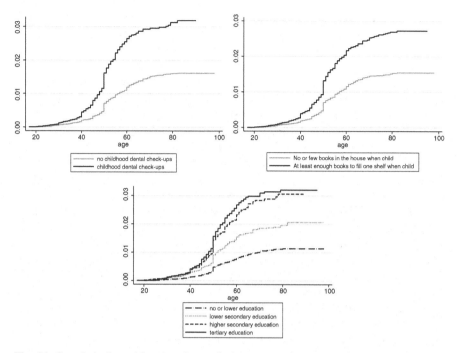

Fig. 6.1 Cumulative hazard functions for starting mammography screening in Belgium, by dental check-ups and cultural capital during childhood, and education (Nelson-Aalen estimates)

2006), childhood conditions seem to play a substantial role in engagement in preventive health behavior during later life and in the accumulation of cultural health capital.

Other forms of cultural capital have become increasingly important within the framework of cultural health capital theory and health lifestyle theory. A measurement of cultural capital in the childhood household (number of books) and a traditional measurement in adulthood (education) could be included. The former is an indicator of objectivized cultural capital in Bourdieu's framework (1986) and is considered to be a powerful proxy for the educational, social, and economic background in early life (Schutz et al. 2008). Figure 6.1 illustrates its significant association with mammography screening (p < 0.001). However, the advantage of cultural capital during childhood (number of books) does not persist after controlling for adulthood social position in the multivariate models. Education is considered as a form of institutionalized cultural capital. It is a distinct aspect of socioeconomic status, as it involves essential problem-solving skills and learned effectiveness, which enable people to control their lives, including health (Mirowsky and Ross 2003). Its decisive role for preventive health habits, such as mammography screening, is well-established (Stirbu et al. 2007). The significant association with education (p < 0.001, see Fig. 6.1) remains crucial, with an increased hazard for mammography screening for tertiary-educated women compared with their lesser-educated counterparts. The effects are even stronger than those for wealth, which suggests that individual competences have indeed become increasingly important.

Principle 2: Timing of Outcomes

Life course researchers are particularly interested in the "social patterns in the timing, duration, spacing and order of events and roles" (Elder and Rockwell 1979, p. 2). Attention is paid to how certain transitions or events can produce different effects depending on their timing within the life course (George 1993). For example, the consequences of the Great Depression were different for older and younger children (Elder 1974). In addition, in life course epidemiology the notions of timing and duration are central to the three main models for the association between early life circumstances and later life: the latency, pathway, and accumulation models (Graham 2002).

By contrast, the temporal dimension of preventive behaviors has been generally ignored in both empirical research (Spadea et al. 2010) and medical sociological theory (Missinne et al. 2014). This is somewhat unfortunate, as the effectiveness of care depends upon a *timely initiation of* preventive care or check-ups and upon its *regular* use. As a result of the focus on rates of illness-related health care use in the Andersen's framework (1983) and the dominant use of cross-sectional study designs, questions about (preventive) health care use are formulated along the lines of: "during the last xx months/years, have you consulted a specialist/GP/dentist/had a mammogram ?". This design and this question wording render it impossible to scrutinize both the timeliness and regularity of preventive behavior. To capture a regular pattern of care, the perception of a 'usual source of care' (e.g. "is there a particular doctor you usually go to when ill, or for advice about health?") is also often used. However, this type of measurement also fails to adequately capture periodic behavior and even the preventive nature of a visit (Newman and Gift 1992).

Timely detection of breast cancer is crucial given that the stage of illness (or tumor size) at diagnosis is strongly linked to survival (Elmore et al. 2005). Therefore, the Council of the European Union recommends that screening programs target women aged 50 to 69 years of age (von Karsa et al. 2008), who are at the highest risk of breast cancer. Age is generally regarded as a control or a confounding variable, or is used as a proxy for 'need' for general health care use (Van der Heyden et al. 2003), preventive health care use (e.g. Jusot et al. 2011), and for mammography screening (e.g. Duport and Ancelle-Park 2006; Wübker 2012). In addition, the *regularity* of preventive habits is recommended. For example, a two-year interval is recommended for mammography screening (European Commission 2003), six months for dental check-ups (Riley et al. 2013) and targeted groups should be given a flu vaccination every year.

In the discussion concerning the social gradient, the temporal dimension should also be included. It is possible that socioeconomic inequalities are partly manifested in both the regularity and the timeliness of preventive health care use, in addition to the probability of ever engaging in it (Missinne et al. 2014). For example, health insurance data has shown that in Belgium, the dropout rate for two-yearly mammography screening is higher among women who benefit from preferential reimbursement (Fabri et al. 2010). Higher-educated groups might be more future oriented and more willing to commit to a long-term goal, such as prevention (Mirowsky and Ross 2003; Wübker 2012). Accordingly, it is possible that cultural health capital includes knowledge or competencies that enable the timely and regular use of preventive health care.

The way the SHARELIFE investigates mammography screening includes both notions of temporality and regularity. The question, *"In which year* did you start having mammograms *regularly?"* was given to all women who answered yes to the question "Have you ever had mammograms regularly over the course of several years?" This retrospective information allows us to gain insight into two important questions relating to the timeliness of mammography screening. The first question relates to the age differences that are often reported for mammography screening. Empirical studies generally report lower engagement in screening among older women (Wübker 2012), but confusion remains substantial (Jepson et al. 2000). The dominant question wording renders it impossible to know whether age differences reflect 'true' age effects or whether they act as proxies for period effects.[4] The latter is very probable, as knowledge about – and policy initiatives concerning – breast cancer and mammography screening have changed considerably in Europe during recent decades (Fisher et al. 2008). To this end, an explorative approach has been followed. Five birth cohorts from 1910 to after 1949 in ten-year intervals were constructed and the Kaplan-Meier graphs were tabulated for the 13 European countries that took part in the SHARELIFE (see Fig. 6.2 for three examples; for details see Missinne and Bracke 2014). The results do indeed suggest substantial period effects. In all countries, earlier birth cohorts overall engage less in screening. Figure 6.2 show that the hazard function for each earlier birth cohort is lower at all ages, except for Sweden. Very similar age trajectories can be observed for each cohort, suggesting no 'true' age effects. The cross-national comparative approach aids in framing these period effects within the context of national screening policies, which have already been empirically linked to the large country-differences in mammography screening (Wübker 2014), illustrated in Fig. 6.4. I will return to this point when elaborating on principle 4. In addition, country-specific deviations can be related to features of national screening policies, again suggesting strong period effects. For example, the coinciding hazards of the two most recent cohorts, as well as an additional increase at the age of 40, can be traced back to the early implementation of a national screening program in 1986, which targets women from the age of 40 in 65 % of Swedish counties. In Belgium, women are invited to participate from the age of 50. In Greece, the absence of a sudden increase indeed

---

[4]Glenn (1976) called statistical attempts to separate age, period and, cohort effects "a futile quest" (for an elaboration, see Glenn 2003). Therefore, I have followed his suggestion to use a more informal approach.

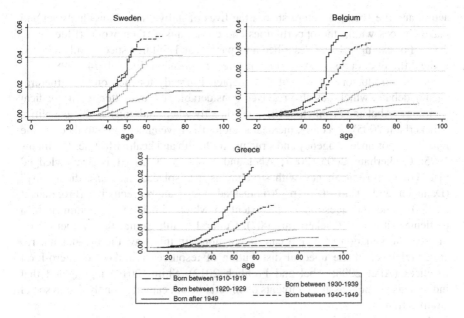

Fig. 6.2 Cumulative hazard function for mammography screening initiation in Sweden, Belgium, and Greece per 10-year birth cohort (Nelson-Aalen estimates)

reflects the absence of a national program (for an overview of screening policies, see von Karsa et al. 2008).

Next, the hypothesis that socioeconomic inequalities could also be manifested in the timeliness of the take-up of mammography screening was tested. Returning to Fig. 6.1 and focusing on the specific age trajectories, an increase of screening around the recommended age of 50 is notable for all social groups. These age trajectories do not differ according to socioeconomic indicators for either childhood (Fig. 6.1) or adulthood (Fig. 6.1). Accordingly, in line with what studies have traditionally assumed, socioeconomic inequalities seem to be manifested in Belgium as a lower probability of ever having a mammogram, rather than in the late commencement of screening. This finding should be interpreted in the light of the relatively small age range for which screening is recommended. The discussion about timeliness should therefore not be closed. For example, for preventive services that begin far more early in life, such as dental check-ups, timeliness might reveal clearer socioeconomic inequalities in preventive health care.

Principle 3: Agency Versus Structure Debate

The principle of agency stresses that individuals are not passive recipients. Encapsulated in life course research is the question of how the interplay between individual action and the social structure shapes the lives of individuals. Individuals act and make choices within the opportunities and constraints of their world (Elder et al. 2003). For example, Elder described how parents and children successfully adapted to the difficult circumstances during the Great Depression (Elder 1974, 1998).

In the introductory section of this chapter, I already touched on the structure-agency debate, which has also received considerable research attention in medical sociology (Abel and Frohlich 2012), most directly when studying health inequalities (Cockerham 2005). Recently, medical sociologists have endeavored to theorize the *relative* importance of agency and structure for health and health lifestyles (Williams 1995; Cockerham 2005, 2007; Abel and Frohlich 2012). It is acknowledged that "counterposing agency with structure is a misplaced and false dichotomy" (Dannefer and Daub 2009, p. 20). Instead, they can be recursive (Frohlich et al. 2001) and the question is the extent to which either one is dominant in a particular situation (Cockerham 2007). Cultural health capital theory focuses on the specific situation of health care interactions. In this way, the broader macro-structural level of the unequal distribution of resources is linked to micro-level practices (Abel 2008; Abel and Frohlich 2012). Shim (2010) highlighted that individuals are not passive recipients of cultural health capital strongly tied to social stratification.

Another way to gain insight into the structure-agency debate is by focusing on the different socialization contexts socially-mobile individuals are confronted with over their life course. Each social position largely determines the 'life chances' of individuals at that time and these positions constitute the structuring forces of 'life choices' (agency) on health lifestyles (Cockerham 2005). The weight that Bourdieu attributed to childhood experiences in the formation of the habitus, has often been critiqued (Daenekindt and Roose 2013). Social mobility research parallels this idea by addressing the multiple contexts of socialization, each with its own health-related practices. Socialization continues into adulthood, when individuals are confronted with new experiences (Ryder 1965) and other significant network members become important for health behaviors (Christakis and Fowler 2007), for example marital partners (see the principle of linked lives). Social mobility research can gain insights into the development of health lifestyles by scrutinizing the relative impact of the social position in childhood versus the prevailing social position.

Using the example of mammography screening has two advantages when study-ing the health behavior of socially-mobile individuals. First, it is only recommended from the age of 50 onwards (WHO 2013), when social mobility processes are likely to have been actualized. Therefore, this type of health behavior is not likely to affect the course of social mobility. In most studies, such a process of reversed causality cannot be ruled out and hampers causal interpretations of the effect of social mobility (Claussen et al. 2005). Second, it is very unlikely that mammography screening is related to the event and the accompanying stress of social mobility itself, as has been suggested for health-compromising behaviors such as alcohol use or dietary patterns (Karvonen et al. 1999).

Diagonal Reference Models (DRMs) were designed in particular to study the effects of social mobility and enable estimation of the relative impact of the social position of origin and the social position of destination. The screening behavior of socially-immobile individuals is taken as the reference points, as they represent the core of each social stratum. Therefore, their health-related behavior is considered characteristic for that social position. Consequently, the health behavior of socially-mobile individuals is modeled as a function of the characteristic behavior of immobile individuals from the social position of origin and of destination (for an outline of the empirical strategy, see Daenekindt and Roose 2013; for examples in health research, see Monden and de Graaf 2012). These models were applied to the Belgian sample of the SHARELIFE to test three hypotheses: (i) health behavior is, in line with Bourdieu, predominantly shaped by the primary socialization context: the social position of *origin*; (ii) the health behavior of socially mobile individuals is predominantly associated with the social position of *destination*; and (iii) the *maximization hypothesis* considers whether the experience of upward social mobility differs from that of downward social mobility. The results showed that the take-up of mammography screening by both upwardly and downwardly mobile individuals reflects the patterns of the women in their prevailing social position. Therefore, empirical support is only found for the second hypothesis. This points to the situational nature of mammography screening, which is also highlighted in the empirical example outlined in the next principle. However, it does not necessarily contradict our findings that childhood socioeconomic conditions are crucial in the development of cultural health capital (principle 1). The data limited us to considering only occupational mobility, which is regrettable given that the role of cultural capital in particular, such as education, has been seen as increasingly important.

Principle 4: Linked Lives

With its principle of linked lives, the life course perspective highlights that individual lives are lived interdependently in a network of shared relationships (Elder et al. 2003). Because experiences are shared, the relevance of various social events and transitions is widened (Heinz and Kruger 2001). These interpersonal experiences are also located within a specific historical time and place that can impact upon these micro-level settings (Elder et al. 2003).

Research on preventive health care and health care in general has focused too much on the individual in isolation. Andersen's (1970, 1995) heuristic model, focuses on how individual need, socioeconomic and demographic characteristics, and individual health beliefs are related to health services use. However, seeking professional care is often not the result of an individual decision, but of an interactive process (Pescosolido 1992). Recently, Umberson and colleagues (2010) drew explicitly on the life course perspective to provide a theoretical framework to unfold the mechanisms underlying the relationship between social ties and health behavior, including preventive health care use and treatment attendance. Predominantly, the focus is on the presumed beneficial effect of marriage. Health-related social control theories propose that partners try to influence and regulate each other's health behavior in order to keep their partners healthy (Lewis et al. 2006; Umberson 1992). However, the universal protective nature of marriage has been challenged (Carr and Springer 2010). Again, the discussion is hindered by the wide use of cross-sectional designs, which make it impossible to discern to what extent the effects attributed to marriage can also be ascribed to premarital health habits and premarital socioeconomic conditions (Meyler et al. 2007). Individual lives are not unwritten pages at the time of marriage. As outlined in the life-span development principle, conditions earlier in life are crucial to the development of health behavior. Although marital partners are the most important and powerful source of influence in a person's adult life, parents are predominant during childhood (Umberson 1992), and also influence socialization into healthy behaviors (Cardol et al. 2005).

In Missinne et al. (2013), we hypothesized that cumulative life course advantages or disadvantages accumulate at the household level and will be greater than at the individual level. Partners provide each other with information and norms on health behavior (Thomas 2011). Therefore, it can be expected that (un)favorable socioeconomic conditions for either partner in childhood will impact on health behavior in later life. Assortative mating can exacerbate these effects and generate systematic divergences over the life course, as contented by cumulative advantage theory (DiPrete and Eirich 2006). Cultural health capital theory might benefit from the explicit inclusion of the notion of linked lives. To elaborate on how capital is acquired and accumulates over time, it is important to understand the role of the childhood and adult preventive health behaviors of both partners.

The dyadic nature of the SHARE and SHARELIFE enabled scrutinizing the influence of the childhood preventive health care behavior of both wives and husbands on the initiation of mammography screening for a sample of Belgian women (N = 734). Figure 6.3 show the Kaplan-Meier graphs for the married women

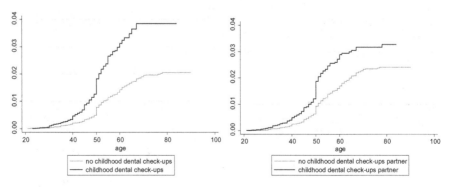

Fig. 6.3 Cumulative hazard functions for the initiation of mammography screening, by childhood dental check-ups of the women and their partners (Nelson-Aalen estimates)

in our sample. As in Fig. 6.1, childhood preventive behavior seems to impact on mammography screening many years later in life ($p < 0.001$). However, what is new is the significant effect of the partner's preventive behavior ($p < 0.001$). Again, the complementary log-log models show that the latter association persists after controlling for the characteristics of the women (number of books during childhood, childhood and lifelong dental check-ups, educational level), the characteristics of the men (childhood and lifelong dental check-ups, educational level), and household wealth. More precisely, the hazard for mammography screening in later life is 25 % higher for women whose husband went regularly for dental check-ups as a child. The results suggest that the cultural health capital of both partners impacts on women's preventive health care use and show the importance of the contextualization of preventive health care use within the family.

Principle 5: Principle of Time and Place

This principle refers to the fact that the life of every individual is embedded in and shaped by a certain historical context and place (Elder et al. 2003). Historical change can impact on an individual's life. It can also engender cohort effects when it alters the lives of successive birth cohorts, and period effects when the effect is more uniform across these cohorts (Elder 1994). The different aftermath of World War II in Europe than in the United States, illustrates that historical events might impact differently across regions or nations (Elder et al. 2003). To translate this idea into empirical practice, life course researchers urge us to expand the scope from national studies, the results of which can be challenged as being too context specific, into international comparative studies (Billari 2009; Blane et al. 2007). This has now become possible in Europe with the advent of some large-scale research projects that have collected life course data which is fully internationally comparative, such as the SHARE.

Although the cross-national comparative approach is well established in health (e.g. Mackenbach 2012) and health care research (e.g. Devaux 2013), it is still upcoming in preventive health care research (Jusot et al. 2011). However, the existing studies have already revealed substantial cross-national variation in preventive health care habits, including mammography screening (e.g. Wübker 2014). An important question now relates to which institutional differences are the driving forces behind this cross-national variation (Blane et al. 2007). For mammography screening, it seems that general (health care) indicators (such as health care expenditure, number of physicians, and gross domestic product) do not matter (Jusot et al. 2011), but that the country-specific characteristics of mammography screening policies should be focused upon (Wübker 2014).

However, the life course perspective encourages us also to incorporate how these institutional factors change over time and how this can potentially interplay with individual development (Elder et al. 2003, p. 11). During the last few decades,

European health care systems have been the subject of almost continuous policy reforms. Many of these reforms have been ad hoc interventions aimed at containing rising expenditure on health care (Mossialos 1997). Further, the specific policies on mammography screening have seen a substantial evolution. For example, in Belgium the first initiatives were taken in 1975 (Van Oyen and Verellen 1994), but it was not until 2001 that the national screening program was actually implemented. Countries also differ greatly with regard to this evolution. National coverage had already been achieved in Sweden in 1997 (Schopper and de Wolf 2009), while Poland (Bastos et al. 2010) and Denmark (Schopper and de Wolf 2009) first implemented their national program about a decade later. Cultural health capital theory and health lifestyle theory would benefit from including this notion of time and place. Studying how preventive health care use is affected by the implementations of or changes to policies, might shed light on the strength of the association between cultural health capital and preventive health behavior, as well as on how cultural health capital is acquired and accumulates over time.

In addition to the careful specification of cohort and period effects in the complementary log-log models, I have incorporated this principle more explicitly by combining a cross-national and a longitudinal approach. Figure 6.2 also serves here as an illustration. Figure 6.4 shows the strong variation in the commencement with regular mammography screenings between the 13 European countries that participated in the SHARELIFE. The cumulative hazard is lowest in Denmark and highest in Sweden. It is remarkable that these extremes are both in the Northern European region, which is generally considered as universally the best performing with regard to health, due to relatively generous and universal welfare provision (Mackenbach 2012).

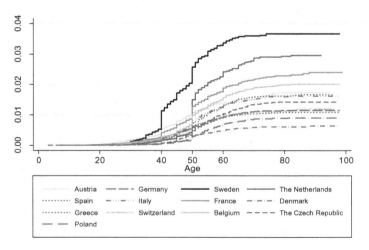

Fig. 6.4 Cumulative hazard function for mammography screening initiation in 13 European countries (Nelson-Aalen estimates)

Conclusion

I have argued that a better understanding of the social roots of preventive health-related behavior can be gained by combining recent theory formation on preventive health care use with insights from theoretical approaches that have traditionally developed outside the domain of health (care), but which show substantial analogies, specifically here a life course perspective. The example of mammography screening is used to illustrate how each of the five principles of the life course perspective raises new questions that can advance the debate substantially. It is important to note that methodological advancements can also be made. Besides the time-issues discussed in the principle of timing, the longitudinal design allows for the correct time ordering of the conditions. Time ordering is often obscured in health care research, as need for health care is almost always defined by means of questions about prevailing health (at the time of the interview), while items on (preventive) health care use the previous week, month, or year as the time framework. This has hampered conclusions on health care inequalities until now, as research has been predominantly based on cross-sectional designs.

The long-term and developmental perspective of the life course highlights the need to shed further light on which conditions at what life stages contribute to the accumulation of cultural health capital. The results of the first (Missinne et al. 2014) and second study (Missinne et al. 2013) suggest that childhood is a critical period in the development of preventive health behavior. They are in line with a fully path-dependent cumulative advantage process, which implies that the effect of socioeconomic conditions early in life has continuing influences on later life outcomes, even when a person's later socioeconomic position is accounted for (DiPrete and Eirich 2006; Willson et al. 2007). It would be insightful to distinguish further between childhood and adolescence, as well as different periods in adulthood life. Moreover, preventive health care research might benefit from considering the life course perspective's additional focus on the length of exposure (duration) to certain social or health conditions. For example, cumulative exposure models (Willson et al. 2007) propose that effects of social mobility can differ according to the amount of time spent in the different social positions (Bartley and Plewis 2007). Therefore, it would be interesting if surveys could include the age at which individuals moved up or down the social ladder. The notion of timeliness brings about the question of the extent to which age differences in other forms of preventive health are attributable to 'true age effects' or to cohort and period effects, as in the case of mammography screening. In addition to timely initiation, socioeconomic inequality research should move beyond a focus on a snapshot on preventive health behaviors and include their continuous or regular use.

The results also illustrate the importance of contextualizing preventive health care habits within the social network, as suggested by the linked lives principle. They suggest that the cultural health capital of both partners accumulates at the marriage level and impacts on women's preventive health care use. What about other important network members? In older age, friends and offspring are also important agents of social control in addition to partners (Lewis and Butterfield 2007). Physicians are also 'significant others' whose roles deserve further attention (Daalman and Elder 2007). Studies have repeatedly shown that even in health care interactions, socioeconomic inequalities exist. For example, it has been reported that more-deprived individuals receive a lower quality of care (Hall and Dornan 1990), spend less time with a doctor (Videau et al. 2010) and receive less information (Willems et al. 2005). Sociological explanations for these divergences are scarce (Willems et al. 2005), but important insights could be derived from the observation that patients in a higher socioeconomic position secure more information from doctors, through effective expressiveness and assertiveness (Verlinde et al. 2012). This active stance precisely constitutes the underlying idea for Shim (2010) developing how cultural health capital may shape the content and tone of patient-provider interactions. The life course perspective highlights that we should extend all these questions beyond the individual level and include the societal processes that shape and reshape the dynamics of inequality that underlie these preventive health care inequalities (Graham 2002). The example of mammography screening illustrates that the role of national policies can be elucidated both by cross-country comparisons and through the study of changes within a single country over time.

A lack of (longitudinal) data and methodological difficulties are only some of the reasons why many of these questions have remained unexplored. At least as important is to keep the underlying theoretical premises in mind. Both life course research and medical sociological theory are particularly well-suited to move beyond the agency-oriented and short-term perspective, which is still dominant in preventive health care research. The life course not only provides a longer-term view and includes the broader societal context, but also stresses that research should be inter-disciplinary, given that inequalities can proliferate across different life domains (Graham 2002).

References

Abel, T. (2008). Cultural capital and social inequality in health. *Journal of Epidemiology and Community Health, 62*, 1–5.
Abel, T., & Frohlich, K. L. (2012). Capitals and capabilities: Linking structure and agency to reduce health inequalities. *Social Science & Medicine*. doi:10.1016/j.socscimed.2011.10.028:236–244.
Andersen, R. M. (1995). Revisiting the behavioral-model and access to medical-care – Does It matter. *Journal of Health and Social Behavior, 36*, 1–10.
Andersen, R. M., Smedby, B., & Anderson, O. W. (1970). *Medical care use in Sweden and the united states – A comparative analysis of systems and behavior*. Chicago: Centre for Health Administration Studies, University of Chicago.

Bartley, M., & Plewis, I. (2007). Increasing social mobility: An effective policy to reduce health inequalities. *Journal of the Royal Statistical Society Series A-Statistics in Society, 170*, 469–481.

Bastos, J., Peleteiro, B., Gouveia, J., Coleman, M. P., & Lunet, N. (2010). The state of the art of cancer control in 30 European countries in 2008. *International Journal of Cancer, 126*, 2700–2715.

Becker, M. H., & Maiman, L. A. (1975). Sociobehavioral determinants of compliance with health and medical care recommendations. *Medical Care, 13*, 10–24.

Billari, F. C. (2009). The life course is coming of age. *Advances in Life Course Research, 14*, 83–86.

Blane, D. (1999). The life course, the social gradient and health. In M. Marmot & R. Wilkinson (Eds.), *Social determinants of health* (pp. 64–80). Oxford: Oxford University Press.

Blane, D. (2008). Social causes of health and disease. *British Journal of Sociology, 59*, 588–589.

Blane, D., Netuveli, G., & Stone, J. (2007). The development of life course epidemiology. *Revue D Epidémiologie et de Santé Publique, 55*, 31–38.

Bogenhold, D. (2001). Social inequality and the sociology of life style – Material and cultural aspects of social stratification. *American Journal of Economics and Sociology, 60*, 829–847.

Bourdieu, P. (1984). *Distinction – A social critique of the judgement of taste.* New York: Routledge.

Bourdieu, P. (1986). The forms of capital. In J. Richardson (Ed.), *Handbook of theory and research for the sociology of education* (pp. 241–258). New York: Greenwood.

Brandt, M., Deindl, C., & Hank, K. (2011). *Tracing the origins of successful aging: The role of childhood conditions and societal context.* MEA discussion paper no. 237–11. Available at SSRN: http://ssrn.com/abstract=1763129

Cardol, M., Groenewegen, P. P., de Bakker, D. H., Spreeuwenberg, P., van Dijk, L., & van den Bosch, W. (2005). Shared help seeking behaviour within families: A retrospective cohort study. *British Medical Journal, 330*, 882–884B.

Carr, D., & Springer, K. W. (2010). Advances in families and health research in the 21st century. *Journal of Marriage and Family, 72*, 743–761.

Christakis, N. A., & Fowler, J. H. (2007). The spread of obesity in a large social network over 32 years. *New England Journal of Medicine, 357*, 370–379.

Clark, T. N., & Lipset, S. M. (2001). Are social classes dying? In T. N. Clark & S. M. Lipset (Eds.), *The breakdown of class politics: A debate on post-industrial stratification* (pp. 39–54). Baltimore: The Johns Hopkins University Press.

Claussen, B., Smits, J., Naess, O., & Smith, G. D. (2005). Intragenerational mobility and mortality in Oslo: Social selection versus social causation. *Social Science & Medicine, 61*, 2513–2520.

Cockerham, W. C. (2000). The sociology of health behavior and health lifestyles. In C. E. Bird, P. Conrad, & A. M. Fremont (Eds.), *Handbook of medical sociology* (pp. 159–172). Upper Saddle River: Prentice-Hall.

Cockerham, W. C. (2005). Health lifestyle theory and the convergence of agency and structure. *Journal of Health and Social Behavior, 46*, 51–67.

Cockerham, W. C. (2007). *Social causes of health and disease.* Cambridge: Polity Press.

Daalman, T., & Elder, G. H. (2007). Family medicine and the life course paradigm. *The Journal of the American Board of Family Medicine, 20*(1), 85–92.

Daenekindt, S., & Roose, H. (2013). Cultural chameleons: Social mobility and cultural practices in private and public sphere. *Acta Sociologica, 56*, 309–324.

Dannefer, D., & Daub, A. (2009). Extending the interrogation: Life span, life course, and the constitution of human aging. *Advances in Life Course Research, 14*(1–2), 15–27.

Devaux, M. (2013). Income-related inequalities and inequities in health care services utilisation in 18 selected OECD countries. *European Journal of Health Economics..* doi:10.1007/s10198-013-0546-4.

DiPrete, T., & Eirich, G. (2006). Cumulative advantage as a mechanisms for inequality: A review of theoretical and empirical developments. *Annual Review of Sociology, 32*, 271–300.

Donovan, J. E., Jessor, R., & Costa, F. M. (1993). Structure of health-enhancing behavior in adolescence – A latent-variable approach. *Journal of Health and Social Behavior, 34*(4), 346–362.

Dubbin, L. A., Chang, J. S., & Shim, J. K. (2013). Cultural health capital and the interactional dynamics of patient-centered care. *Social Science & Medicine, 93*, 113–120.

Due, P., Krolner, R., Rasmussen, M., Andersen, A., Damsgaard, M. T., Graham, H., & Holstein, B. E. (2011). Pathways and mechanisms in adolescence contribute to adult health inequalities. *Scandinavian Journal of Public Health, 39*, 62–78.

Duport, N., & Ancelle-Park, R. (2006). Do socio-demographic factors influence mammography use of French women? Analysis of a French cross-sectional survey. *European Journal of Cancer Prevention, 15*, 219–224.

Elder, G. H. (1974). *Children of the great depression: Social change in life experiences*. Chicago: University of Chicago Press.

Elder, G. H. (1994). Time, human agency, and social-change - perspectives on the life course. *Social Psychology Quarterly, 57*, 4–15.

Elder, G. H., Jr. (1998). The life course as developmental theory. *Child Development, 69*, 1–12.

Elder, G. H., & Rockwell, R. C. (1979). Life course and human-development – Ecological perspective. *International Journal of Behavioral Development, 2*, 1–21.

Elder, G. H., Johnson, M. K., & Crosnoe, R. (2003). The emergence and development of life course theory. In J. T. Mortimer & M. J. Shanahan (Eds.), *Handbook of the life course* (pp. 3–19). New York: Kluwer.

Elmore, J. G., Armstrong, K., Lehman, C. D., & Fletcher, S. W. (2005). Screening for breast cancer. *JAMA, 293*, 1245–1256.

European Commission. (2003). *Council recommendations on cancer screening*. http://ec.europa.eu. Accessed 20 May 2012.

Fabri, V., Remacle, A., & Boutsen, M. (2010). *Programme de Dépistage du Cancer du Sein: Comparaison des trois premiers tours 2002–2003, 2004–2005 et 2006–2007 (rapport 7)*. Bruxelles: Aence Intermualiste (IMA).

Ferlay, J., Parkin, D. M., & Steliarova-Foucher, E. (2010). Estimates of cancer incidence and mortality in Europe in 2008. *European Journal of Cancer, 46*, 765–781.

Ferlay, J., Steliarova-Foucher, E., Lortet-Tieulent, J., Rosso, S., Coebergh, J. W., Comber, H., Forman, D., & Bray, F. (2013). Cancer incidence and mortality patterns in Europe: Estimates for 40 countries in 2012. *European Journal of Cancer, 49*, 1374–1403.

Fishbein, M., & Ajzen, I. (1975). *Belief, attitude, intervention, and behavior: An introduction to theory and research*. Reading: Addison-Wesley.

Fisher, B., Redmond, C. K., & Fisher, E. R. (2008). Evolution of knowledge related to breast cancer heterogeneity: A 25-year retrospective. *Journal of Clinical Oncology, 26*(13), 2068–2071.

Frohlich, K. L., Corin, E., & Potvin, L. (2001). A theoretical proposal for the relationship between context and disease. *Sociology of Health & Illness, 23*, 776–797.

Gamoran, A., & Mare, R. D. (1989). Secondary-school tracking and educational-inequality – Compensation, reinforcement, or neutrality. *American Journal of Sociology, 94*, 1146–1183.

Gangl, M. (2004). Welfare states and the scar effects of unemployment: A comparative analysis of the United States and West Germany. *American Journal of Sociology, 109*, 1319–1364.

George, L. K. (1993). Sociological perspectives on life transitions. *Annual Review of Sociology, 19*, 353–373.

Glenn, N. D. (1976). Cohort analysts futile quest – Statistical attempts to separate age, period and cohort effects. *American Sociological Review, 41*, 900–904.

Glenn, N. D. (2003). Distinguishing age, period, and cohort effects. In J. T. Mortimer & M. J. Shanahan (Eds.), *Handbook of the life course* (pp. 465–476). New York: Kluwer Academic/Plenum Publishers.

Gotzsche, P. C., & Nielsen, M. (2009). Screening for breast cancer with mammography. *Cochrane Database of Systematic Reviews, 4*, Artn Cd001877.

Graham, H. (2002). Building an inter-disciplinary science of health inequalities: The example of lifecourse research. *Social Science & Medicine, 55*, 2005–2016.

Hakama, M., Coleman, M. P., Alexe, D. M., & Auvinen, A. (2008). Cancer screening: Evidence and practice in Europe 2008. *European Journal of Cancer, 44*, 1404–1413.

Halfon, N., & Hochstein, M. (2002). Life course health development: An integrated framework for developing health, policy, and research. *Milbank Q, 80*, 433–479. iii.

Hall, J. A., & Dornan, M. C. (1990). Patient sociodemographic characteristics as predictors of satisfaction with medical-care – A meta-analysis. *Social Science & Medicine, 30*, 811–818.

Hayward, M. D., & Gorman, B. K. (2004). The long arm of childhood: The influence of early-life social conditions on men's mortality. *Demography, 41*, 87–107.

Heinz, W. R., & Krüger, H. (2001). Life course: Innovations and challenges for social research. *Current Sociology, 49*(2), 29–45.

Jemal, A. (2011). Global cancer statistics. *CA: A Cancer Journal for Clinicians, 61*, 69–90.

Jepson, R., Clegg, A., Forbes, C., Lewis, R., Snowden, A., & Kleijnen, J. (2000). The determinants of screening uptake and interventions for increasing uptake: A systematic review. *Health Technology Assessment, 4*, 1–133.

Jusot, J. F., Or, Z., & Sirven, N. (2011). Variations in preventive care utilisation in Europe. *European Journal of Ageing.* doi:10.1007/s10433-011-0211-7.

Karvonen, S., Rimpela, A. H., & Rimpela, M. K. (1999). Social mobility and health related behaviours in young people. *Journal of Epidemiology and Community Health, 53*, 211–217.

Kuh, D., Ben-Shlomo, Y., Lynch, J., Hallqvist, J., & Power, C. (2003). Life course epidemiology. *Journal of Epidemiology and Community Health, 57*(10), 778–783.

Kuh, D., Power, C., Blane, D., & Bartley, M. (2004). Socioeconomic pathways between childhood and adult health. In D. Kuh & Y. Ben Shlomo (Eds.), *A life course approach to chronic disease epidemiology* (pp. 371–395). Oxford: Oxford University Press.

Lau, R. R., Quadrel, M. J., & Hartman, K. A. (1990). Development and change of young-adults preventive health beliefs and behavior – Influence from parents and peers. *Journal of Health and Social Behavior, 31*, 240–259.

Lewis, M. A., & Butterfield, R. M. (2007). Social control in marital relationships: Effect of one's partner on health behaviors. *Journal of Applied Social Psychology, 37*(2), 298–319.

Lewis, M. A., McBride, C. M., Pollak, K. I., Puleo, E., Butterfield, R. M., & Emmons, K. M. (2006). Understanding health behavior change among couples: An interdependence and communal coping approach. *Social Science & Medicine, 62*, 1369–1380.

Mackenbach, J. P. (2012). The persistence of health inequalities in modern welfare states: The explanation of a paradox. *Social Science & Medicine, 75*, 761–769.

Meyler, D., Stimpson, J. P., & Peek, M. K. (2007). Health concordance within couples: A systematic review. *Social Science & Medicine, 64*, 2297–2310.

Mirowsky, J., & Ross, C. E. (2003). *Education, social status, and health.* New York: de Gruyter, Inc.

Missinne, S., & Bracke, P. (2014). Age differences in mammography screening reconsidered: Life course trajectories in 13 European countries. *European Journal of Public Health.* doi:10.1093/eurpub/cku077.

Missinne, S., Colman, E., & Bracke, P. (2013). Spousal influence on mammography screening: A life course perspective. *Social Science & Medicine, 98*, 63–70.

Missinne, S., Neels, K., & Bracke, P. (2014). Reconsidering inequalities in preventive health care: An application of cultural health capital theory and the life course perspective. *Sociology of Health & Illness, 36*(8), 1259–1275.

Monden, C. W., & de Graaf, N. D. (2012). The importance of father's and own education for self-assessed health across Europe: An east-west divide? *Sociology of Health & Illness, 35*, 977–992.

Mossialos, E. (1997). Citizens' views on health care systems in the 15 member states of the European Union. *Health Economics, 6*, 109–116.

Newman, J. F., & Gift, H. C. (1992). Regular pattern of preventive dental services – A measure of access. *Social Science and Medicine, 35*, 997–1001.

Pescosolido, B. A. (1992). Beyond rational choice – The social dynamics of how people seek help. *American Journal of Sociology, 97*, 1096–1138.

Phelan, J. C., Link, B. G., Diez-Roux, A., Kawachi, I., & Levin, B. (2004). "Fundamental causes" of social inequalities in mortality: A test of the theory. *Journal of Health and Social Behavior, 45*, 265–285.

Rajaram, S. S., & Rashidi, A. (1998). Minority women and breast cancer screening: The role of cultural explanatory models. *Preventive Medicine, 27*, 757–764.

Riley, P., Worthington, H. V., Clarkson, J. E., & Beirne, P. V. (2013). Recall intervals for oral health in primary care patients (review). *The Cochrane Library*. doi:10.1002/14651858.

Ryder, N. B. (1965). The cohort as a concept in the study of social-change. *American Sociological Review, 30*, 843–861.

Schafer, M. H., Ferraro, K. F., & Mustillo, S. A. (2011). Children of misfortune: Early adversity and cumulative inequality in perceived life trajectories. *American Journal of Sociology, 116*, 1053–1091.

Schopper, D., & de Wolf, C. (2009). How effective are breast cancer screening programmes by mammography? Review of the current evidence. *European Journal of Cancer, 45*, 1916–1923.

Schutz, G., Ursprung, H. W., & Wossmann, L. (2008). Education policy and equality of opportunity. *Kyklos, 61*, 279–308.

Shim, J. K. (2010). Cultural health capital: A theoretical approach to understanding health care interactions and the dynamics of unequal treatment. *Journal of Health and Social Behavior, 51*, 1–15.

Singh-Manoux, A., & Marmot, M. (2005). Role of socialization in explaining social inequalities in health. *Social Science & Medicine, 60*, 2129–2133.

Spadea, T., Bellini, S., Kunst, A., Stirbu, I., & Costa, G. (2010). The impact of interventions to improve attendance in female cancer screening among lower socioeconomic groups: A review. *Preventive Medicine, 50*, 159–164.

Stirbu, I., Kunst, A., Mielck, A., & Mackenbach, J. P. (2007). *Educational inequalities in utilization of preventive services among elderly in Europe*. Rotterdam: Department of Public Health.

Thomas, P. A. (2011). Trajectories of social engagement and limitations in late life. *Journal of Health and Social Behavior, 52*, 430–443.

Tinsley, B. J., Markey, C. N., Ericksen, A. J., Ortiz, R. V., & Kwasman, A. (2002). Health promotion for parents. In M. H. Bornstein (Ed.), *Handbook of parenting: Practical issues in parenting* (Vol. 5, pp. 311–328). London: Lawrence Erlbaum Associates.

Umberson, D. (1992). Gender, marital-status and the social-control of health behavior. *Social Science & Medicine, 34*, 907–917.

Umberson, D., Crosnoe, R., & Reczek, C. (2010). Social relationships and health behavior across the life course. *Annual Review of Sociology, 36*(36), 139–157.

Van der Heyden, J. H. A., Demarest, S., Tafforeau, J., & Van Oyen, H. (2003). Socio-economic differences in the utilisation of health services in Belgium. *Health Policy, 65*, 153–165.

van Doorslaer, E., Masseria, C., & Koolman, X. (2006). Inequalities in access to medical care by income in developed countries. *Canadian Medical Association Journal, 174*, 177–183.

Van Oyen, H., & Verellen, W. (1994). Breast cancer screening in the Flemish region, Belgium. *European Journal of Cancer Prevention, 3*, 7–12.

Verlinde, E., Delaender, N., DeMaesschalck, S., Deveugele, M., & Willems, S. (2012). The social gradient in doctor-patient communication. *International Journal of Equity in Health, 11*, 12.

Videau, Y., Saliba-Serre, B., Paraponaris, A., & Ventelou, B. (2010). Why patients of low socioeconomic status with mental health problems have shorter consultations with general practitioners. *Journal of Health Services Research & Policy, 15*(2), 76–81.

von Karsa, L., Anttila, A., Ronco, G., Ponti, A., Malila, N., Arbyn, M., et al. (2008). *Cancer Screening in the European Union. Report on the implementation of the Council Recommendation on cancer screening*. Luxembourg: European Communities.

Weber, M. (1922/1978). *Economy and society* (Vol. 1). Berkeley, California: University of California Press.

WHO. (2013). *Breast cancer: Prevention and control*. http://www.who.int/cancer/detection/breastcancer/en/. Accessed 8 Sept 2013.

Wickrama, K. A. S., Conger, R. D., Wallace, L. E., & Elder, G. H. (1999). The intergenerational transmission of health-risk behaviors: Adolescent lifestyles and gender moderating effects. *Journal of Health and Social Behavior, 40*(3), 258–272.

Willems, S., De Maesschalck, S., Deveugele, M., Derese, A., & De Maeseneer, J. (2005). Socio-economic status of the patient and doctor-patient communication: Does it make a difference? *Patient Education and Counseling, 56*, 139–146.

Williams, S. J. (1995). Theorizing class, health and life-styles – Can Bourdieu help Us. *Sociology of Health & Illness, 17*(5), 577–604.

Willson, A. E., Shuey, K. M., & Elder, G. H. (2007). Cumulative advantage processes as mechanisms of inequality in life course health. *American Journal of Sociology, 112*, 1886–1924.

Wu, L. L. (2003). Event history models for life course analysis. In J. T. Mortimer & M. J. Shanahan (Eds.), *Handbook of the life course* (pp. 477–502). New York: Kluwer.

Wübker, A. (2012). Who gets a mammogram amongst European women aged 50–69 years? *Health Economics Review, 2*, 1–13.

Wübker, A. (2014). Explaining variations in breast cancer screening across European countries. *The European Journal of Health Economics, 15*(5), 497–514.

Youlden, D. R., Cramb, S. M., Dunn, N. A., Muller, J. M., Pyke, C. M., & Baade, P. D. (2012). The descriptive epidemiology of female breast cancer: An international comparison of screening, incidence, survival and mortality. *Cancer Epidemiology, 36*, 237–248.

Chapter 7
Inter-Cohort Variation in the Consequences of U.S. Military Service for Men's Mid- to Late-Life Body Mass Index Trajectories

Janet M. Wilmoth, Andrew S. London, and Christine L. Himes

Obesity, as measured by body mass index (BMI), is considered one of the most pressing public health concerns in the United States (U.S. Department of Health and Human Services 2001). Although obesity rates have recently stabilized, the prevalence of obesity in the adult population increased for all sex and age groups between 1980 and 2010 (Flegal et al. 1998, 2010; Ogden et al. 2012). In the most recent data, 35.7 % of adults in the United States—over 78 million people—were considered obese (Ogden et al. 2012). Since obesity is associated with a variety of health problems, most notably diabetes (Narayan et al. 2007), and with increased disability at older ages (Himes 2000), understanding the mechanisms by which subgroups of the population do and do not gain weight as they age is important.

The obesity epidemic in the United States coincided with a substantial shift in men's participation in the U.S. military. In the middle of the twentieth century, military service early in adulthood was a normative part of the life course for the majority of men in the United States (Hogan 1981). However, in 1973, the U.S. military ended conscription and moved into the current All-Volunteer Force era. Relative to the participation rates of men from early-twentieth-century birth cohorts, which peaked around 80 % for those who served during World War II (Hogan 1981), rates of military service among young adults in more recent cohorts have dropped substantially. Nevertheless, military service remains a salient pathway to adulthood for many young adults in the United States (Wilmoth and London 2013; Wolf et al. 2013). If military service influences weight and weight gain across the life course, then the passage of cohorts through the age structure during historical

J.M. Wilmoth (✉) • A.S. London
Department of Sociology and Aging Studies Institute, Syracuse University, Syracuse, NY, USA
e-mail: jwilmoth@maxwell.syr.edu

C.L. Himes
Lewis College of Human Sciences, Illinois Institute of Technology, Chicago, IL, USA

© The Author(s) 2015   133
C. Burton-Jeangros et al. (eds.), *A Life Course Perspective on Health Trajectories and Transitions*, Life Course Research and Social Policies 4,
DOI 10.1007/978-3-319-20484-0_7

periods characterized by different levels of early-adulthood engagement in military service could contribute to population-level changes in age-specific obesity rates.

At the individual-level, military service is a potential source of variation in BMI outcomes that is often overlooked in the extant literature. A growing body of life course research examines the health consequences of service in the U.S. military in different historical periods (Dobkin and Shabani 2009; Elder et al. 1997; MacLean 2013; Teachman 2011; Whyman et al. 2011; Wilmoth et al. 2010). However, until recently (Teachman and Tedrow 2013), researchers have not focused much attention on veteran status differences in BMI or whether military service affects changes in BMI over the life course. One consequence of this omission is that there is little evidence regarding the importance of veteran status relative to other individual-level characteristics that are commonly examined in the BMI literature, such as childhood disadvantage, race/ethnicity, socioeconomic status, and health behaviors. Given that the military carefully screens the health and body weight of those who enlist or are inducted into service (Poston et al. 2005; Wolf et al. 2013), and early-life weight is a strong predictor of later-life weight (Ferraro et al. 2003), veterans might be expected to weigh less and have a lower prevalence of obesity than non-veterans. However, somewhat paradoxically, previous research shows that body weight among veterans is generally similar to or higher than body weight among non-veterans (Almond et al. 2008; Wang et al. 2005; Teachman and Tedrow 2013).

A well-controlled, comparative examination of BMI trajectories by veteran status has the potential to inform our understanding of the veteran status-weight paradox and shed light on the early- and later-life factors that influence change in weight over the life course more broadly. Therefore, in this chapter, we examine the relationship between service in the U.S. military and men's BMI trajectories in mid- to late-life. We are particularly interested in comparing older veterans and non-veterans within successive cohorts who were subjected to specific historical circumstances in terms of periods of war and peace, as well as dietary practices and norms regarding daily physical activity. Our approach allows us to isolate the effect of U.S. military service for given cohorts from the broader health-related trends that have driven increases in BMI in the U.S. population over time. It also provides insight into how following particular pathways in the transition to adulthood can have enduring implications for development and the influence of historical time on life course outcomes, both of which are central features of the life course perspective (Wilmoth and London 2013).

Military Service and Physical Health

There are various mechanisms by which military service in early adulthood could have effects on later-life physical health outcomes, for better or worse (Wilmoth and London 2013). In theory, military service may be associated with better health because of selection, directly beneficial effects of military service, or the indirect effects of military service on mid- to later-life health-related outcomes. Because of pre-induction or -enlistment screening that blocks the entry of persons with observable health problems from joining the military (Sackett and Mayer 2006), veterans may, on average, be in better health than non-veterans in earlier periods of the adult life course. Additionally, during war, active-duty personnel are screened for combat readiness, which could contribute to a "healthy warrior" effect among war-service veterans. Beyond selection, the intense physical training and fitness required of military personnel may produce health benefits or encourage life-long participation in exercise, while the resources to which veterans have access through the U.S. Department of Veterans Affairs can indirectly affect health by shaping a range of health-related outcomes, such as educational attainment (Bennett and McDonald 2013), employment and earnings (Kleykamp 2013), and marriage and family integration (Burland and Lundquist 2013). In addition, military service can operate as a positive turning point in the life course, particularly for individuals from disadvantaged socioeconomic backgrounds, because it "knifes off" prior negative influences and creates a "bridging environment" that provides access to educational, training, and health care resources (Elder 1986, 1987; London and Wilmoth 2006; Sampson and Laub 1996).

Although there are good theoretical reasons to consider, and some empirical evidence supporting, the potential benefits of military service for physical health, the bulk of the available evidence documents negative health and disability consequences. Service-related factors that could negatively impact health outcomes include: training accidents and over-training injuries; hazardous work assignments; deployment to locales with infectious disease conditions that are detrimental to health; financial strains and other stressors related to separation from family and work; the distribution of subsidized tobacco products by the military; and placement in environments that are conducive to substance use or heavy drinking (Bedard and Deschênes 2006; Clipp and Elder 1996; Elder and Clipp 1988, 1989; Elder et al. 2009). In addition, wartime service often involves combat exposure, which increases the risk of short-term injury and long-term disability (Elder et al. 1997; MacLean 2010, 2013), physical and mental health problems (Elder et al. 2009; Vogt et al. 2004), and later-life mortality (Elder et al. 2009). Thus, wartime service should have a more negative impact on later-life health than non-war service.

There is a substantial literature on the physical health of veterans that documents a high prevalence of poor health, functional limitation, and disability (Aldwin et al. 1994; Beebe 1975; Centers for Disease Control 1998; Keehn 1980; Schnurr et al. 2000). Service members and veterans who were deployed to war zones are more likely to report ill health and chronic fatigue, gastrointestinal diseases, skin disorders, and chronic pain (Armed Forces Health Surveillance Center 2009; Institute of Medicine 2008). While providing important data on the health of veterans that is useful for some policy and planning purposes, this literature usually does not directly examine differences between veterans and non-veterans, compare veterans with and without wartime service, or attempt to determine the extent to which service during particular historical periods or wars has different effects on later-life health.

In addition to the research that focuses on veterans only, there is comparative evidence based on data from the general population that documents the enduring effects of military service on health and disability. Veterans who served during wartime, particularly World War II (WWII) and the Korean War, experience steeper later-life health declines than non-veterans (Wilmoth et al. 2010). Veterans—especially combat veterans (MacLean 2010)—also have higher rates of functional limitations and disabilities than non-veterans (Wilmoth et al. 2010). Compared to non-veterans, Vietnam War veterans are more likely to rate their health as fair or poor, have physical limitations, and be anxious or depressed (Dobkin and Shabani 2009). Similar evidence is derived from studies of more recent veterans. Recent research indicates that at age 40, veterans who served on active duty during the era of the All-Volunteer Force (which began when conscription ended in 1973) report poorer self-rated health, even after controlling for a range of covariates, including socioeconomic status and health behaviors (Teachman 2011). The higher rates of poor health, functional limitation, and disability among veterans during midlife may contribute to health disparities in later life by influencing the economic well-being of veteran families; recent research indicates that households containing disabled veterans experience an increased risk of poverty and material hardship (Heflin et al. 2012; London et al. 2011; Wilmoth et al. 2015).

Military Service and Body Weight

The effects of military service on health status may be related to the underlying effect of military service on specific health behaviors, such as drug and alcohol use, smoking, sleep, diet, and exercise (London et al. 2014; Miech et al. 2013). One specific health risk factor of current interest is obesity, which is indicated by a BMI score of 30.0 or higher (Hsu et al. 2007; Lindquist and Bray 2000). Among active-duty service members, obesity is relatively rare, although it has been increasing. In 2005, approximately 12 % of active-duty military personnel had a BMI score of 30.0 or higher, compared to 5 % of active-duty personnel 10 years earlier (Armed Forces Health Surveillance Center 2009) and about 35 % of all adults in the United States (Ogden et al. 2012). Despite this apparent active-duty advantage, numerous studies have either found that veteran status is unrelated to body size (Almond et al. 2008; Wang et al. 2005) or that veterans are more likely to be obese than non-veterans (Koepsell et al. 2009; Teachman and Tedrow 2013). However, the research that focuses on military service and weight is mostly descriptive, often focuses on veterans only, and generally does not adequately control for early-life factors that select people into military service (Almond et al. 2008; Das et al. 2005; Nelson 2006; Rosenberger et al. 2011; for an exception, see Teachman and Tedrow 2013). Moreover, some studies focus only on users of Veterans Health Administration services (Das et al. 2005; Wang et al. 2005), which is a highly selected and disadvantaged segment of the veteran population.

One recent life course study has contributed substantially to our understanding of the connections between military service and weight gain over the life course. In the era of the All-Volunteer Force, Teachman and Tedrow (2013) argue that eating and exercise patterns are more in balance during the active-duty period than they are during the more-sedentary veteran period. Eating habits established while in the military, when physical activity and caloric demands are relatively high, carry over into civilian life, but activity levels and exercise habits do not carry over to the same extent. As a result, during the transition to civilian life, veterans gain weight and then carry that weight with them as they age. From this perspective, the military is a protective environment to the extent that it encourages physical activity during and after the period of active duty, but is a risk environment to the extent that it encourages eating habits that can lead to weight gain.

The BMI measure is a ratio of weight to height and does not measure body fat directly. Consequently, one possible explanation for why veteran men weigh more than non-veteran men is that they have more muscle mass, resulting in a high BMI score but a low fat-to-lean body mass ratio (Koepsell et al. 2012). Physical training in the military may increase muscle mass, which increases BMI, and high BMI at one point in time generally portends high BMI at a later point in time. Rosenberger et al. (2011) studied veterans of Iraq and Afghanistan and reported that higher initial BMI was associated with greater increases in BMI over 6 years for each of the five BMI trajectory groups they identified. Koepsell et al. (2012) reported that among NHANES subjects veterans had higher weight than non-veterans by self-report and direct measurement of BMI, waist-stature ratio, and waist circumference, but were less likely than non-veterans to have 35+ % body fat. One implication of viewing the military as a potentially protective environment that encourages physical activity is that the establishment of early-life patterns of exercise and muscle development may be particularly beneficial to individuals who are genetically predisposed toward obesity.

With the exception of Teachman and Tedrow (2013), past studies of veteran status and body size have looked only at a point in time rather than examining the trajectory of body weight change with age. Body weight for an individual is not stable over time. Cross-sectional studies show that body weight increases through adulthood until about age 65, and then declines (Flegal et al. 1998). Longitudinal studies show mixed results with respect to the factors influencing weight gain. The long-term trajectory of BMI over adulthood shows a largely linear increase with age for both men and women (Botoseneanu and Liang 2011), although weight gain appears to slow with age (He and Baker 2004). The well-documented secular increase in obesity prevalence is reflected in longitudinal studies; the BMI trajectories of younger cohorts are steeper than those of the older cohorts examined (Clarke et al. 2009).

In the United States context, findings are mixed with respect to identifying the influence of various factors on the rate of BMI change with age. Most studies indicate that women have higher rates of weight gain with age than men (Clarke et al. 2009; He and Baker 2004; Mujahid et al. 2005; Walsemann and Ailshire 2011), although some find no gender difference (Botoseneanu and Liang 2011). Race is related to BMI trajectories, but its effects vary by gender. Black and Hispanic men have higher rates of weight gain (Clarke et al. 2009); however, Botoseneanu and Liang (2011) find that non-Hispanic Black men gain less weight over time than White men even though they enter middle age with higher BMI. Examinations of body weight trajectories in the Alameda County Study indicate that early-life factors, particularly educational attainment, are important in determining the trajectory of weight change over age, especially for women (Baltrus et al. 2005). However, other studies have found no effect of education or income on weight gain (He and Baker 2004).

The Current Investigation

BMI is an important health indicator that changes with age and may be shaped in important ways by prior military service. While a high proportion of older men in the United States served in the military, to date, there has been no longitudinal, population-representative study of veteran status differences in men's mid- to late-life BMI trajectories reported in the literature. As such, the potential influence of prior military service on weight change among older men remains largely hidden. In our research, we examine veteran status differences in mid- to late-life BMI trajectories for cohorts of men born in the United States during the first half of the twentieth century. Our primary research questions are: (1) How is veteran status related to BMI in mid- to late-life?; (2) Do veterans have different BMI trajectories than non-veterans, controlling for early- and mid- to late-life characteristics?; and (3) Do the BMI trajectories of veterans and non-veterans vary depending on birth cohort?

Methods

Data

This study uses data from the 1992 to 2010 longitudinal Assets and Health Dynamics among the Oldest Old (AHEAD), Health and Retirement Study (HRS), and RAND HRS files (henceforth HRS). The analytic sample for this study includes 12,277 men born between 1895 and 1956. During the 18 years of the study, these men contributed 68,483 observations to the person-period file that we use to estimate the conditional growth curve models described below. We limit the analysis to men because less than 1 % (135) of the 14,491 women in the HRS served in the military.

Measures

Dependent Variable The dependent variable for this analysis is *BMI*, which is equal to weight in kilograms/height in meters squared. Both height and weight are self-reported.

Table 7.1 Birth cohorts by years turned 18 and age ranges in 1992 and 2010

Cohort birth years	Years turned 18 (historical period)	Age range in 1992	Age range in 2010
<1929	<1947 (WWII)	64 and older	82 and older
1929–1936	1947–1954 (Post-WWII/Korean War)	56–63	74–81
1937–1945	1955–1963 (Cold War)	47–55	65–73
1946–1956	1964–1974 (Vietnam War)	36–46	54–64

Notes: The 1992 HRS included subjects ages 51–61 who were born between 1931 and 1941. Older subjects in our analysis were initially recruited into AHEAD, which collected data from subjects ages 70 and older in 1993. The HRS and AHEAD were merged in 1998 at the same time additional birth cohorts were recruited into the study. HRS age-eligible subjects are over the age of 50 at the time of entry into the study. For details regarding the HRS study design see http://hrsonline.isr. umich.edu/sitedocs/DesignHistory.pdf.

Independent Variables There are two focal independent variables in this analysis: veteran status and birth cohort. The HRS contains a retrospective self-report of "active military service," not including service in the military reserves. We used these data to construct a binary *veteran status* measure (yes = 1).

In order to facilitate comparisons between veterans and non-veterans who came of age during different time periods, we constructed a measure of *birth cohort* that takes into account when respondents turned age 18, which is approximately when they became eligible to serve in the military, regardless of whether they actually entered the military. We used a conservative approach in that we assumed that men who turned 18 in the year a conflict officially ended were primarily eligible for service in the subsequent time period (e.g., veteran men who turned 18 in 1955 would have primarily served after the end of the Korean War). Some veteran men who turned 18 in the year a conflict ended might have served during that conflict right before it ended or as the conflict was winding down; however, the majority of their multi-year service would have been in the subsequent time period.

We created four cohorts as shown in Table 7.1: the first was born prior to 1929 and turned 18 before the end of WWII in 1946; the second was born from 1929 to 1936 and turned 18 from 1947 to 1954, during the years after WWII and during the Korean War; the third was born from 1937 to 1945 and turned age 18 between 1955 and 1963, during the Cold War; and the fourth was born from 1946 to 1956 and turned age 18 between 1964 and 1974, during the Vietnam War. It is important to keep in mind these cohorts represent the time period in which respondents turned age 18 and therefore became eligible for service, not the specific period of service among veterans. Although the men in these cohorts were eligible to serve in the military when they turned 18, some of the veterans in the sample could have served during subsequent or multiple time periods. Those who served exclusively during the Cold War would not have been subjected to combat. Additionally, given that more military personnel serve in support roles than combat roles, it is likely that the majority of those who served during WWII, the Korean War, and the Vietnam War also did not experience direct combat; however, we are unable to determine service in war zones or combat exposure due to data limitations.

It should be noted that the youngest subjects entered the HRS later in the study period and therefore contributed fewer person-period observations to the analysis. This is due to the design of the HRS, which initially included subjects who were ages 51–61 in 1992, who were born between 1931 and 1941, and its companion study, the AHEAD, which collected data from subjects ages 70 and older in 1993, who were born before 1924. Individuals born from 1924 to 1930 and after 1941 were not included in the HRS until it was merged with the AHEAD and moved to a steady-state design in 1998. At that point, two cohorts—one born 1924–1930 and the other born from 1942 to 1947—were added. Since 1998, additional new cohorts have been added every 6 years (Health and Retirement Study 2008).

Control and Potentially Mediating Variables The analysis includes a broad range of control and potentially mediating variables, which prior research indicates are associated with both veteran status and BMI. The first set of control variables are retrospectively reported early-life characteristics that occurred prior to military service: race/ethnicity, early-life socioeconomic disadvantage, and early-life health. Race/ethnicity includes *non-Hispanic White* (reference), *non-Hispanic Black*, *non-Hispanic other race*, and *Hispanic* (of any race). Early-life socioeconomic disadvantage is an indexed scale, which is comprised of four dichotomously coded retrospective childhood variables: mother's education and father's education (*<8 years* = 1; *≥8 years* = 0); father's occupation when the respondent was age 16 (*unskilled manual* = 1, *non-manual, skilled, and professional* = 0); and overall family SES from birth to age 16 (*poor* = 1, *not poor, including the family was "pretty well off financially," "about average," and "it varied"* = 0). Per the procedure outlined in Wilmoth et al. (2010), respondents missing on any of these four variables were assigned to the zero category for that variable, which is a conservative approach to dealing with missing data because that category represents greater advantage and misclassification would bias toward the null. We summed these four variables and divided by the number of items answered to create an early-life disadvantage scale that ranges from 0 to 1, with higher values indicating more disadvantage. Because a relatively large proportion of respondents had missing values on at least one early-life disadvantage item, which is due primarily to father's absence or attrition prior to the 1998 survey when these questions were asked for the first time, we also include a variable in the models that is equal to one for all individuals for whom at least one of these variables was missing and set to zero. Additionally, the analysis includes a measure of health from birth to age 16 years that measures *poor health* and *missing* relative to good health (reference).

The other variables, which reference mid- to late-life characteristics that potentially mediate the relationship between military service and BMI, are measured many years after military service has ended. All of these mid- to late-life variables, except education, are time-varying across the 18-year study period. Marital status includes four categories: *married* (reference), *never married*, *divorced/separated*, and *widowed*. Education is measured at entry into the HRS and includes *high school or less* (reference), *some college or college graduate*, and *more than college*. Household income is measured in dollars. Labor force status is recoded as a binary variable (*in the labor force* = 1). Two health behaviors are measured dichotomously: ever smoked cigarettes (*yes* = 1) and currently drinks alcohol (*yes* = 1).

Finally, we include three methodological controls. These are binary variables measuring ever had a proxy interview (*yes* = 1), dropping out of the study (*yes* = 1), and dying during the 18-year time span of the study (*yes* = 1).

Analysis Plan

After describing the sample, we estimate conditional growth curve models using the person-period file described above and the PROC MIXED procedure in SAS. In all of these trajectory analyses, we define time in terms of chronological age (as opposed to study duration) because we are interested in modeling age-related changes in BMI. The grand mean age for all sample members, which is equal to 67 years, is used to center age.

Models include terms for age and age squared to test for nonlinearity in the relationship between age and BMI. Additionally, we include terms that interact age and age squared with the veteran status and cohort measures to account for potential nonlinearity in the slope that estimates age-related changes in BMI in relation to our focal variables. The models control hierarchically for early-life and mid- to late-life characteristics, as well as methodological controls for proxy response, attrition, and death over the study period, although the coefficients for those controls are not shown (full models are available upon request). We focus on interpreting the coefficients for the effect of veteran status and cohort membership on BMI at the mean age of 67 years, and the effect of veteran status and cohort membership on age-related change in BMI. Positive coefficients indicate that men who are veterans or in a particular cohort have higher BMI relative to the reference group, whereas negative coefficients indicate the opposite.

To facilitate the interpretation of the fully-specified model, we present predicted age-related BMI trajectories by birth cohort and veteran status. The predicted values represent men with the following characteristics: non-Hispanic White; mean early-life disadvantage; good early-life health; high school graduate; out of the labor force; mean household income; married; never smoked; current non-drinker; never had a proxy interview; not lost to follow up; and did not die during the study period. Predicted values are only presented for the age ranges over which the birth cohorts are observed during the study period, which are shown in Table 7.1. The figure only presents predicted values at age 50 and older because the men must have been at least 50 to be eligible for inclusion in the HRS.

Results

Sample Description

Table 7.2 presents descriptive statistics overall and by veteran status. As seen in Table 7.2, the characteristics of veterans and non-veterans differ substantially. Overall, the mean BMI is 27.4, with veterans having slightly, but significantly, lower BMI than non-veterans (27.34 versus 27.49). The mean age of the sample is 67, but veterans are significantly older than non-veterans. The sample is fairly evenly distributed across the first three birth cohorts, with each containing less than one-third of the sample; as expected due to the design of the HRS (see discussion in Methods), the youngest cohort has a substantially smaller percentage (11 %). Consistent with the very high rates of participation in the military in and around WWII, veterans are over-represented among the oldest two cohorts, while non-veterans have relatively higher representation in the younger two cohorts.

There are significant differences between veterans and non-veterans with respect to the early-life controls. Veterans are significantly more likely than non-veterans to be non-Hispanic White (85 % versus 69 %), which is expected on the basis of the policies that prevailed prior to the end of World War II (see Lutz 2013). Interestingly, the mean childhood disadvantage index is lower among veterans than non-veterans, but, as expected, a smaller percentage of veterans report having had poor childhood health.

There are also significant veteran status differences in the potentially mediating variables. Education levels are higher among veterans, with 35 % having attended or graduated from college (compared to 22 % among non-veterans). Veterans are more likely to be currently out of the labor force and have mean household incomes that are significantly lower than non-veterans. Veterans are slightly more likely to be currently married (81 %) than non-veterans (79 %). In addition, veterans are significantly more likely than non-veterans to have ever smoked (76 % versus 66 %) and to currently drink alcohol (60 % versus 55 %).

Finally, veterans and non-veterans differ with respect to the methodological controls. During the study period, veterans are less likely than non-veterans to have had a proxy report (19 % versus 27 %) or be lost to follow-up (16 % versus 18 %), but are somewhat more likely to have died during the course of the study (24 % versus 23 %).

BMI Trajectories in Later Life

Table 7.3 presents four models predicting BMI. Model 1, which only includes age, age squared, and veteran status, indicates that veterans have significantly lower BMI than non-veterans at the mean-centered age of 67. In addition, as expected, for all men, BMI decreases at an increasing rate with age.

Table 7.2 Total sample characteristics by veteran status[a]

	Total sample		Non-veteran		Veteran		
	%	Mean	%	Mean	%	Mean	p
Variable							
BMI		27.40		27.49		27.34	***
Age (*in years*)		67.00		65.62		68.15	***
Veteran							
Yes	54.52						
No	45.48						
Birth cohort							
<1929	27.17		21.27		32.09		***
1929–1936	29.46		25.00		33.17		
1937–1945	32.19		38.35		27.06		
1946–1956	11.18		15.38		7.68		
Race/ethnicity							
White	77.13		69.54		85.02		***
Black	12.63		17.23	16.56	9.35		
Other	2.14		3.00		1.42		
Hispanic	8.10		12.77		4.21		
Childhood disadvantage index (*0–1*)	0.34			0.37		0.32	***
Poor childhood health							
Yes	4.37		5.41		3.50		***
No	95.63		94.59		96.50		
Education							
High school or less	58.05		64.81		52.41		***
Attended/graduated college	29.26		22.48		34.92		
More than college	12.69		12.71		12.67		
Labor force participation							
Yes	31.97		36.72		28.01		***
No	68.03		63.28		71.99		
Household income (*in $1,000*)	62.50			64.94		60.47	*
Marital status							
Married/partnered	80.46		79.32		81.43		***
Divorced/separated	8.37		8.94		7.89		
Widowed	8.29		8.06		8.48		
Never married	2.88		3.68		2.20		
Ever smoked							
Yes	71.43		66.20		75.79		***
No	28.57		33.80		24.21		
Currently drinks alcohol							
Yes	57.66		54.51		60.29		***
No	42.34		45.49		39.71		

(continued)

Table 7.2 (continued)

	Total sample		Non-veteran		Veteran		
	%	Mean	%	Mean	%	Mean	p
Proxy report							
Yes	23.17		27.34		19.69		***
No	76.83		72.66		80.31		
Lost to follow-up							
Yes	17.29		18.47		16.31		***
No	82.71		81.53		83.69		
Died							
Yes	23.70		22.81		24.44		***
No	76.30		77.19		75.56		

Significance: $*p < 0.05$; $**p < 0.01$; $***p < 0.001$
[a]Data are un-weighted

Model 2 controls for birth cohort. Interestingly, the coefficient for veteran status is now positive and marginally significant, indicating that, at the mean-centered age of 67, veterans have higher BMI than non-veterans once cohort is taken into account. This is because older cohorts, which have lower BMI than younger cohorts, include an over-representation of veterans. Compared to the cohort that came of age during WWII, each subsequent cohort has significantly higher BMI. It is noteworthy that the coefficients for the cohorts are quite large and increase by approximately 1 point with each successive cohort. Compared to the <1929 cohort (that turned 18 during WWII), the 1929–1926 cohort (that turned 18 during the post-WWII/Korean War period) has a BMI that is 1.24 points higher, the 1937–1945 cohort (that turned 18 during the Cold War) has a BMI that is 2.16 points higher, and the 1946–1956 cohort (that turned age 18 during the Vietnam War) has a BMI that is 3.11 points higher. With cohort controlled, the sign on the age coefficient becomes positive, while the age-squared coefficient remains negative.

Model 3 includes terms that estimate the age-related trajectories by veteran status and cohort. The coefficient for veteran remains positive, but is now significant, and the cohort coefficients continue to be relatively large and positive. In this model, the coefficients for age and age-squared are both negative, although only the age-squared term is significant. The coefficients that indicate the age-based trajectories for veterans reveal that, compared to non-veterans, BMI increases more rapidly with age for veterans (this difference is marginally significant). In addition, compared to the <1929 cohort, the other three cohorts experience more rapid increases in weight gain with age.

Model 4 adds controls for early- and mid- to late-life characteristics, as well as methodological controls for proxy interviews, loss to follow-up, and death. The results remain essentially the same as reported for Model 3. BMI decreases at an increasing rate with age. Veterans continue to have higher BMI at the mean-centered age, although the coefficient is marginally significant. The three younger cohorts have significantly higher BMI at the mean-centered age, compared to the WWII

Table 7.3 Growth curve models predicting BMI trajectories

Fixed effects	Model 1[a]	Model 2[b]	Model 3[c]	Model 4[d]
Total sample				
Intercept	27.7747	26.1949***	26.3522***	27.2601***
	(0.061)	(0.093)	(0.127)	(0.170)
Veteran	−0.2042*	0.1527+	0.1985*	0.1759+
	(0.079)	(0.079)	(0.089)	(0.091)
Age	−0.0228***	0.0078**	−0.0029	0.0038
	(0.002)	(0.003)	(0.015)	(0.015)
Age^2	−0.0044***	−0.0043***	−0.0045***	−0.0047***
	(0.001)	(0.000)	(0.001)	(0.001)
1929–1936 birth cohort		1.2636***	1.0057***	0.8917***
		(0.110)	(0.139)	(0.142)
1937–1945 birth cohort		2.1551***	1.9501***	1.7836***
		(0.114)	(0.140)	(0.148)
1946–1956 birth cohort		3.1134***	3.1229***	2.9791***
		(0.133)	(0.240)	(0.253)
Age*veteran			0.0083+	0.0068
			(0.004)	(0.004)
Age^2*veteran			−0.0005	−0.0005+
			(0.000)	(0.000)
Age*1929–1936 birth cohort			0.0119	0.0005
			(0.015)	(0.015)
Age^2*1929–1936 birth cohort			0.0016*	0.0015*
			(0.001)	(0.001)
Age*1937–1945 birth cohort			0.0420**	0.0339*
			(0.016)	(0.016)
Age^2*1937–1945 birth cohort			0.0033***	0.0032***
			(0.001)	(0.001)
Age*1946–1956 birth cohort			0.0616	0.0473
			(0.038)	(0.038)
Age^2*1946–1956 birth cohort			0.0037*	0.0033+
			(0.002)	(0.002)
−2 log likelihood	309,112.8	308,510.8	308,264.9	308,134.3
AIC	309,134.8	308,538.8	308,338.9	308,216.3
BIC	309,216.8	308,643.1	308,614.6	308,521.8
Number of observations	68,483	68,483	68,483	68,483
Number of cases	12,722	12,722	12,722	12,722

Notes: Significance levels: $+p < 0.10$; $*p < 0.05$; $**p < 0.01$; $***p < 0.001$
[a]Model only includes age and veteran status variables
[b]Model controls for birth cohort
[c]Model includes age-related trajectories by veteran status and birth cohort
[d]Model controls for race/ethnicity, early-life socioeconomic disadvantage, early-life health, education, income, labor force participation, marital status, smoking, drinking, proxy interview, lost to follow up, and death during the study period

cohort. However, the age*veteran coefficient is no longer significant, but the age-squared*veteran coefficient is marginally significant and negative, indicating that veteran BMI decreases at an increasing rate with age. For the three younger birth cohorts, BMI increases at an increasing rate with age.

Supplemental analysis suggests that the veteran status results are sensitive to model specification. While the cohort coefficients are consistently significant and large, the significance of the veteran coefficient meets the $p < 0.05$ standard in some models, but is marginally significant in other models. For example, the supplemental model that only included controls for early-life characteristics found that veteran status is marginally significant. This suggests early-life characteristics that are related to selection into military service explain some of the relationship between veteran status and mid- to late-life BMI. When we add the potentially mediating mid- to late-life variables, the veteran status coefficient becomes significant at conventional levels. This indicates some of the effect of veteran status on BMI operates through mid- to late-life characteristics that are related to BMI. In the fully-specified Model 4 shown in Table 7.3, veteran status once again becomes marginally significant when the methodological controls are included. Overall, these supplemental analyses consistently show that veterans have slightly higher BMI and less rapid weight gain trajectories with age, although in some of these models these effects are marginally significant.

Although the coefficients for the covariates are not shown (results available upon request), it is noteworthy that BMI is significantly higher among respondents who currently drink alcohol (compared to those who do not drink alcohol), and significantly lower among respondents who are other race (compared to non-Hispanic Whites), have college or graduate education (compared to those with a high school education or less), are divorced/separated, widowed, or never married (compared to currently married), ever smoked (compared to never smoked), ever had a proxy interview (compared to those who never had a proxy interview), and died during the study period (compared to those who did not die). Childhood disadvantage, childhood health, Black and Hispanic race/ethnicity, and household income are not significant in the fully specified model.

Figure 7.1 presents the age-based BMI trajectories by cohort and veteran status that are based on the fully-specified Model 4 in Table 7.3. The figure demonstrates that, within each cohort, veterans are modestly heavier than non-veterans at every age. Also, the overall pattern of the BMI trajectories for veterans and non-veterans within each cohort is similar, which suggests that military service has a consistent effect on mid- to late-life BMI trajectories regardless of cohort. The observed cross-cohort differences in BMI trajectories are noteworthy, as they are substantially larger than the observed intra-cohort effect of veteran status. Each successive cohort is heavier and appears to exhibit more rapid weight gain early in later-life. The difference in BMI across cohorts at age 65, which is an age at which all of the cohorts were actually observed in the data, is substantial. For example, the predicted BMI at age 65 for the <1929 cohort is just under 27.5, whereas it is nearly 30.5 for the 1946–1956 cohort.

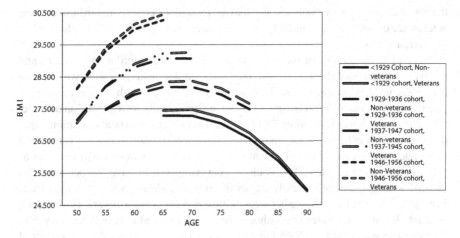

Fig. 7.1 Predicted BMI trajectories by birth cohort and veteran status

Discussion

This research examines whether age-related BMI trajectories among older men vary by veteran status. In order to compare veterans and non-veterans who came of age during different historical periods, we constructed a measure of birth cohort that corresponds to when respondents turned age 18 and became eligible to serve in the military, regardless of whether they actually entered the military. This approach allows us to examine intra-cohort veteran status differences and to account for those who served, respectively, during war and peacetime. While there are many reasons to expect that military service will contribute to lower body weight later in life, we find that veterans have slightly higher BMI than non-veterans and they have similar trajectories of weight change with age. Our key findings emerge across a set of hierarchical models. Without any controls in the models, veterans exhibit lower BMI, on average, than non-veterans. This would support the argument that military service provides protective effects against weight gain over the life course. However, since veterans are over-represented in older cohorts that have lower BMI, on average, the effect of veteran status reverses once cohort is controlled. Once we add controls for early-life characteristics that occur prior to military service, potentially mediating mid- to late-life characteristics, and methodological controls for proxy report, attrition, and death during the study period, the effect of veteran status is small, marginally significant, and positive—within each cohort, veterans are marginally heavier than their non-veteran counterparts. Although the effect of veteran status is small relative to the very large effect of cohort membership, the same can be said for other covariates that have been the focus of other individual-level studies of BMI, such as childhood disadvantage, Black and Hispanic race/ethnicity, and household income. Taken together, our analyses demonstrate the over-riding effect of the secular trend in increased weight across the population—younger cohorts are heavier than older cohorts regardless of their veteran status—and a substantively small but consistent, positive intra-cohort effect of veteran status.

We find the trajectory of weight change with age to be similar for veterans and non-veterans across cohorts. Overall, the predicted age pattern is slow weight gain across age until about age 65–70, followed by more-rapid weight loss at older ages. The two older cohorts, born before 1937, have significantly lower BMI, on average, than the two cohorts born after 1937. These two older cohorts also exhibit rapid declines in BMI in later life. Given that the younger two cohorts have not yet entered these later ages, it remains to be seen how their BMI trajectories will play out as they age into their eighties. The younger cohorts appear to have steeper increases in BMI with age during the early stages of later-life, although direct comparisons in trajectories across these earlier ages with the cohorts born before 1937 cannot be made because the older two cohorts were not observed during their early 50s. Other researchers using the HRS have found similar patterns over the age ranges of actual measurement (ages 51–75), but have not estimated predicted trajectories past that age range (Botoseneanu and Liang 2011; He and Baker 2004; Walsemann and Ailshire 2011).

Each successive cohort is most likely heavier because members of the younger cohorts experienced the well-documented late-twentieth century dietary changes in the United States earlier in their life course, and have lived with those eating patterns for a larger portion of their lives. Around 1970, diets in the United States began to shift toward increased consumption of soft drinks, snack food, and fast food in conjunction with lower consumption of fresh fruits and vegetables; portion size also increased along with total caloric intake, which has fueled the current obesity epidemic (Wang and Beydoun 2007). The youngest cohort in this analysis, which was born from 1946 to 1956, would have been 14–24 in 1970; the oldest cohort, which was born before 1929, would have been over 41 in 1970. Thus, our models demonstrate the cumulative effect of being exposed early in the life course to food consumption patterns that are associated with obesity. This trend towards heavier body size in younger cohorts, despite increases in physical activity, is mirrored in studies of active-duty military personnel (Lindquist and Bray 2000), as well as the general population.

Our research adds to the small body of work examining body size and veteran status. In line with some previous work (Almond et al. 2008; Wang et al. 2005), we find little substantive difference in body weight between veterans and non-veterans within the same cohort, although the estimated effect is marginally significant in the fully-specified model that includes a broad range of potentially mediating variables. In an analysis similar to ours, Teachman and Tedrow (2013) did find an effect of military service on body weight, with veterans being heavier. However, their analysis, based on men born after 1968, looks at a much younger and more recent cohort.

The physical demands and dietary control of military life contribute to an expectation that veterans should have lower body weight than non-veterans. Exercise and dietary habits formed in young adulthood might be expected to carry through to later life, resulting in lower overall weight and slower weight gain. However, our analyses show that the opposite is true. Veterans, if anything, are slightly heavier than their peers who did not experience military service. More-refined measures of current diet and levels of physical activity are needed to determine how these early-life habits change after leaving military service. One possible explanation is that eating habits acquired during active-duty service, when physical activities and caloric demands are high, do not change with exit from active-duty service and the shift to lower levels of physical activity (Teachman and Tedrow 2013). Another possibility is that the exercise and fitness regimes of the military contribute to veteran status differences in lean muscle to fat ratios, with such compositional differences contributing to veteran status differences in BMI and health across the life course (Koepsell et al. 2012).

Our analyses are limited by the constraints of the available data. While we are able to control for several early-life factors that are related to selection into the military and BMI, we do not have measures of early-life body weight. In addition, our measures of current BMI are based on self-reported measures of height and weight rather than on direct measurement. Self-reported BMI tends to be lower than directly measured BMI; however, veterans and non-veterans are similarly likely to under-report (Koepsell et al. 2012). Therefore, BMI is potentially influenced by normative bias, especially at the extreme ends of height and weight distributions. In addition, BMI itself is limited as a measure of obesity since it does not take into account differences in body composition. To the extent that veterans have greater muscle mass relative to body fat, BMI will overstate obesity. The findings might also mask important sources of BMI heterogeneity among veterans. For example, the effect of military service on BMI over the life course may operate through the lingering deleterious outcomes that are experienced by some military personnel who have engaged in combat, such as post-traumatic stress disorder and disabling physical injuries. Conversely, the military requirements for physical fitness might have had enduring positive effects for those who served as non-combat personnel, in particular branches of service, or in the officer ranks. Unfortunately, the HRS data upon which these analyses are based do not contain information about variation in veteran's military service experiences. When such data become available, future studies that examine heterogeneity in military service experiences have the potential to nuance our understanding of the influence of military service on mid- and late-life BMI trajectories.

Despite these limitations, this research contributes to our understanding of the complex ways that military service can impact later-life BMI and health. We are able to compare several cohorts of men who served in the military during different historical periods. We control for many early-, mid-, and late-life characteristics associated with selection into the military and health outcomes. Our finding of large cohort differences confirm other research documenting the secular trend towards increased body size in the general population (Flegal et al. 2010), while our finding of small, positive intra-cohort veteran status differences provides evidence that early-life institutional factors can have enduring effects across the life course. Despite the health habits related to exercise and fitness that are encouraged and enforced by the military, veterans were not protected from the broader social changes driving increases in BMI since the middle of the twentieth century. This finding has implications for policies that attempt to encourage healthy habits related to exercise and fitness in other institutional contexts in which young adults participate—namely higher education and prisons. While exercise promotion might have short-term impacts, it may not have enduring effects in a cultural context of unhealthy dietary practices.

It is not known whether the relationship between BMI and veteran status that we observe in this sample of older adult men in the United States would be found in other countries where the context of military service and trends in BMI differ. Similar to the United States, many older men in countries like England, France, Germany, Italy, Russia, China, and Japan served in the military during the middle of the twentieth century. These countries have also experienced rising BMI among more recent cohorts. Carefully conducted comparisons of cohort-specific BMI trajectories among veterans and non-veterans in other national contexts would enable researchers to determine the importance of military service relative to the influence of cohort membership and other individual-level characteristics, including health behaviors.

If datasets from other countries contain more detailed information about military service experiences, then such additional analyses could begin to identify the service-related factors that contribute to greater weight gain in later life. Until such studies are pursued, much can be learned by studying cross-cohort differences in military service experiences within a given country. For example, obtaining a better understanding how military policies regarding food rations during service and subsidized food in commissaries have varied across time could provide insight into how the food consumption patterns of military personnel and veterans might be different from the civilian non-veteran population in ways that would increase the risk of weight gain. Such research would also have implications for understanding the dietary practices and BMI of those who spend time in other institutional settings, like schools and prisons, which provide a large portion (if not all) of daily caloric intake to their members.

Both cross-national and single-country studies of the relationship between military service and BMI would benefit from employing a life course perspective that conceptualizes mid- to late-life outcomes as being rooted in experiences in childhood and young adulthood, and longitudinal models that capitalize on panel studies with steady state designs that follow successive cohorts as they age. Only then will the influence of military service on later-life health, and health-related outcomes like BMI, be fully understood. More importantly, such studies would advance life course research by providing insight into how specific pathways during the transition to adulthood and unique historical contexts experienced by particular cohorts shape later-life outcomes.

Acknowledgement This work was supported in part by NIH Grant #1R01AG028480-01 (PI: Janet M. Wilmoth).

References

Aldwin, C. M., Levenson, M. R., & Spiro, A., III. (1994). Vulnerability and resilience to combat exposure: Can stress have lifelong effects? *Psychology and Aging, 9*(1), 34–44. doi:10.1037/0882-7974.9.1.34.

Almond, N., Kahawati, L., Kinsinger, L., & Porterfield, D. (2008). Prevalence of overweight and obesity among U.S. military veterans. *Military Medicine, 173*, 544–549. doi:10.7205/MILMED.173.6.544.

Armed Forces Health Surveillance Center. (2009). *Medical surveillance monthly report, 16*(1), 1–28. http://www.dtic.mil/cgi-bin/GetTRDoc?AD=ADA495050&Location=U2&doc=GetTRDoc.pdf

Baltrus, P. T., Lynch, J. W., Everson-Rose, S., Ragthunathan, T. E., & Kaplan, G. A. (2005). Race/ethnicity, life-course socioeconomic position, and body weight trajectories over 34 years: The Alameda County Study. *American Journal of Public Health, 95*, 1595–1601. doi:10.2105/AJPH.2004.046292.

Bedard, K., & Deschênes, O. (2006). The long-term impact of military service on health: Evidence from World War II and Korean War veterans. *American Economic Review, 96*(1), 176–194. doi:10.1257/000282806776157731.

Beebe, G. W. (1975). Follow-up studies of World War II and Korean prisoners. II. Morbidity, disability, and maladjustments. *American Journal of Epidemiology, 101*(5), 400–422.

Bennett, P. R., & McDonald, K. B. (2013). Military service as a pathway to early socioeconomic achievement for disadvantaged groups. In J. M. Wilmoth & A. S. London (Eds.), *Life-course perspectives on military service* (pp. 119–143). New York: Routledge.

Botoseneanu, A., & Liang, J. (2011). Social stratification of body weight trajectory in middle-age and older Americans: Results from a 14-year longitudinal study. *Journal of Aging and Health, 23*, 454–480. doi:10.1177/0898264310385930.

Burland, D., & Lundquist, J. H. (2013). The best years of our lives: Military service and family relationships – a life-course perspective. In J. M. Wilmoth & A. S. London (Eds.), *Life-course perspectives on military service* (pp. 165–184). New York: Routledge.

Centers for Disease Control. (1998). Health status of Vietnam veterans. II. Physical health. *Journal of the American Medical Association, 259*(18), 2708–2714. doi:10.1001/jama.1988.03720180034029.

Clarke, P., O'Malley, P. M., Johnston, L. D., & Schulenberg, J. E. (2009). Social disparities in BMI trajectories across adulthood by gender, race/ethnicity and lifetime socio-economic position: 1986–2004. *International Journal of Epidemiology, 38*, 499–509. doi:10.1093/ije/dyn214.

Clipp, E. C., & Elder, G. H., Jr. (1996). Aging veteran of World War II: Psychiatric and life course insights. In P. E. Ruskin & J. A. Talbott (Eds.), *Aging and posttraumatic stress disorder* (pp. 19–51). Washington, DC: American Psychiatric Association Press.

Das, S. R., Kinsinger, L. S., Yancy, W. S., Wang, A., Ciesco, E., Burdick, M., et al. (2005). Obesity prevalence among veterans at Veterans Affairs medical facilities. *American Journal of Preventive Medicine, 28*(3), 291–294. doi:10.1016/j.amepre.2004.12.007.

Dobkin, C., & Shabani, R. (2009). The health effects of military service: Evidence from the Vietnam draft. *Economic Inquiry, 47*(1), 69–80. doi:10.1111/j.1465-7295.2007.00103.x.

Elder, G. H., Jr. (1986). Military times and turning points in men's lives. *Developmental Psychology, 22*(2), 233–245. doi:10.1037/0012-1649.22.2.233.

Elder, G. H., Jr. (1987). War mobilization and the life course: A cohort of World War II veterans. *Sociological Forum, 2*(3), 449–472. doi:10.1007/BF01106621.

Elder, G. H., Jr., & Clipp, E. C. (1988). Combat experience, comradeship, and psychological health. In J. P. Wilson, Z. Harel, & B. Kahana (Eds.), *Human adaptation to extreme stress: From the Holocaust to Vietnam* (pp. 131–156). New York: Plenum.

Elder, G. H., Jr., & Clipp, E. C. (1989). Combat experience and emotional health: Impairment and resilience. *Journal of Personality, 57*(2), 311–341. doi:10.1111/j.1467-6494.1989.tb00485.x.

Elder, G. H., Jr., Shanahan, M. J., & Clipp, E. C. (1997). Linking combat and physical health: The legacy of World War II in men's lives. *American Journal of Psychiatry, 154*(3), 330–336. doi:10.1176/ajp.154.3.330.

Elder, G. H., Jr., Clipp, E. C., Brown, J. S., Martin, L. R., & Friedman, H. S. (2009). The lifelong mortality risks of World War II experiences. *Research of Aging, 31*(4), 391–412. doi:10.1177/0164027509333447.

Ferraro, K., Thorpe, R., & Wilkinson, J. (2003). The life course of severe obesity: Does childhood overweight matter? *The Journals of Gerontology. Series B, Psychological Sciences and Social Sciences, 58*, S110–S119. doi:10.1093/geronb/58.2.S110.

Flegal, K. M., Carroll, M. D., Kuczmarski, R. J., & Johnson, C. L. (1998). Overweight and obesity in the United States: Prevalence and trends, 1960-1994. *International Journal of Obesity and Related Metabolic Disorders, 22*, 39–47. doi:10.1038/sj.ijo.0800541.

Flegal, K. M., Carroll, M. D., Ogden, C. L., & Curtin, L. R. (2010). Prevalence and trends in obesity among US adults, 1999-2008. *JAMA, 303*, 235–241. doi:10.1001/jama.2009.2014.

He, X. Z., & Baker, D. W. (2004). Changes in weight among a nationally representative cohort of adults aged 51 to 61, 1992 to 2000. *American Journal of Preventive Medicine, 27*, 8–15. doi:10.1016/j.amepre.2004.03.016.

Health and Retirement Study (2008). Sample Evolution: 1992–1998. http://hrsonline.isr.umich.edu/sitedocs/surveydesign.pdf

Heflin, C. M., Wilmoth, J. M., & London, A. S. (2012). Veteran status and material hardship: The moderating influence of disability. *Social Service Review, 86*(1), 119–142. doi:10.1086/665643.

Himes, C. L. (2000). Obesity, disease, and functional impairment in later life. *Demography, 37*, 73–82. doi:10.2307/2648097.

Hogan, D. P. (1981). *Transitions and social change: The early lives of American men.* New York: Academic.

Hsu, L. L., Nevin, R. L., Tobler, S. K., & Rubertone, M. V. (2007). Trends in overweight and obesity among 18-year-old applicants to the U.S. military, 1993-2006. *Journal of Adolescent Health, 41*, 610–612. doi:10.1016/j.jadohealth.2007.07.012.

Institute of Medicine. (2008). *Gulf war and health: volume 6. Physiologic, psychologic, and psychosocial effects of deployment-related stress.* http://www.iom.edu/Reports/2007/Gulf-War-Health-Vol-6-Physiologic-Psychologic-Psychosocial-Effects-Deployment-Related-Stress.aspx

Keehn, R. J. (1980). Follow-up studies of World War II and Korean conflict prisoners. III. Mortality to January 1, 1976. *American Journal of Epidemiology, 111*(2), 194–211.

Kleykamp, M. (2013). Labor market outcomes among veterans and military spouses. In J. M. Wilmoth & A. S. London (Eds.), *Life-course perspectives on military service* (pp. 144–164). New York: Routledge.

Koepsell, T., Forsberg, C., & Littman, A. (2009). Obesity, overweight, and weight control practices in U.S. veterans. *Preventive Medicine, 23*, 521–528. doi:10.1016/j.ypmed.2009.01.008.

Koepsell, T. D., Littman, A. J., & Forsberg, C. W. (2012). Obesity, overweight, and their life course trajectories in veterans and non-veterans. *Obesity, 20*(2), 434–439. doi:10.1038/oby.2011.2.

Lindquist, C. H., & Bray, R. M. (2000). Trends in overweight and physical activity among U.S. military personnel, 1995-1998. *Preventive Medicine, 32*, 57–65. doi:10.1006/pmed.2000.0771.

London, A. S., & Wilmoth, J. M. (2006). Military service and (dis)continuity in the life course: Evidence on disadvantage and mortality from the Health and Retirement Study and the Study of Assets and Health Dynamics among the Oldest-Old. *Research on Aging, 28*(1), 135–159. doi:10.1177/0164027505281572.

London, A. S., Heflin, C. M., & Wilmoth, J. M. (2011). Work-related disability, veteran status, and poverty: Implications for family well-being. *Journal of Poverty, 15*(3), 330–349. doi:10.1080/10875549.2011.589259.

London, A. S., Burgard, S. A., & Wilmoth, J. M. (2014). The influence of veteran status, psychiatric diagnosis, and traumatic brain injury on inadequate sleep. *Journal of Sociology and Social Welfare, 41*(4), 49–67.

Lutz, A. C. (2013). Race-ethnicity and immigration status in the U.S. military. In J. M. Wilmoth & A. S. London (Eds.), *Life-course perspectives on military service* (pp. 68–96). New York: Routledge.

MacLean, A. (2010). The things they carry: Combat, disability, and unemployment among U.S. men. *American Sociological Review, 75*(4), 563–585. doi:10.1177/0003122410374085.

MacLean, A. (2013). A matter of life and death: Military service and health. In J. M. Wilmoth & A. S. London (Eds.), *Life-course perspectives on military service* (pp. 200–220). New York: Routledge.

Miech, R. A., London, A. S., Wilmoth, J. M., & Koester, S. (2013). The effects of the military's antidrug policies over the life course: The case of past-year hallucinogen use. *Substance Use & Misuse, 48*, 837–853. doi:10.3109/10826084.2013.800120.

Mujahid, M. S., Diez Roux, A. V., Borrell, L. N., & Nieto, F. J. (2005). Cross-sectional and longitudinal associations of BMI with socioeconomic characteristics. *Obesity Research, 13*(8), 1412–1421. doi:10.1038/oby.2005.171.

Narayan, K. M., Boyle, J. P., Thompson, T. J., Gregg, E. W., & Williamson, D. F. (2007). Effect of BMI on lifetime risk for diabetes in the U.S. *Diabetes Care, 30*(6), 1562–1566. doi:10.2337/dc06-2544.

Nelson, K. M. (2006). The burden of obesity among a national probability sample of veterans. *Journal of General Internal Medicine, 21*(9), 915–919. doi:10.1007/BF02743137.

Ogden, C. L., Carroll, M. D., Kit, B. K., & Flegal, K. M. (2012). *Prevalence of obesity in the United States, 2009–2010* (NCHS data brief, Vol. 82). Hyattsville: National Center for Health Statistics.

Poston, W. S. C., Haddock, C. K., Peterson, A. L., Vander Weg, M. W., Klesges, R. C., Pinkston, M. M., & DeBon, M. (2005). Comparison of weight status between two cohorts of U.S. Air Force recruits. *Preventive Medicine, 40*, 602–609. doi:10.1016/j.ypmed.2004.09.006.

Rosenberger, P. H., Ning, Y., Brandt, C., Allore, H., & Haskell, S. (2011). BMI trajectory groups in veterans of the Iraq and Afghanistan wars. *Preventive Medicine, 53*(3), 149–154. doi:10.1016/j.ypmed.2011.07.001.

Sackett, P. R., & Mayer, A. S. (Eds.). (2006). *Assessing fitness for military enlistment: Physical, medical, and mental health standards*. Washington, DC: The National Academies Press.

Sampson, R. J., & Laub, J. H. (1996). Socioeconomic achievement in the life course of disadvantaged men: Military service as a turning point, circa 1940-1965. *American Sociological Review, 61*(3), 347–367. doi:10.2307/2096353.

Schnurr, P. P., Spiro, A., III, & Paris, A. H. (2000). Physician-diagnosed medical disorders in relation to PTSD symptoms in older male military veterans. *Health Psychology, 19*(1), 91–97. doi:10.1037/0278-6133.19.1.91.

Teachman, J. (2011). Are veterans healthier? Military service and health at age 40 in the All-Volunteer Force era. *Social Science Research, 40*(1), 326–335. doi:10.1016/j.ssresearch.2010.04.009.

Teachman, J., & Tedrow, L. (2013). Veteran status and body weight: A longitudinal fixed-effects approach. *Population Research and Policy Review, 32*(2), 199–220. doi:10.1007/s11113-012-9262-5.

U.S. Department of Health and Human Services. (2001). *The surgeon general's call to action to prevent and decrease overweight and obesity*. Rockville: US Department of Health and Human Services, Public Health Office, Office of the Surgeon General.

Vogt, D. S., King, D. W., King, L. A., Savarese, V. W., & Suvak, M. K. (2004). War-zone exposure and long-term general life adjustment among Vietnam veterans: Findings from two perspectives. *Journal of Applied Social Psychology, 34*(9), 1797–1824. doi:10.1111/j.1559-1816.2004.tb02586.x.

Walsemann, K. M., & Ailshire, J. A. (2011). BMI trajectories during the transition to older adult-hood: Persistent, widening, or diminishing disparities by ethnicity and education? *Research on Aging, 33*(3), 286–311. doi:10.1177/0164027511399104.

Wang, Y., & Beydoun, M. A. (2007). The obesity epidemic in the United States—Gender, age, socioeconomic, racial/ethnic, and geographic characteristics: A systematic review and meta-regression analysis. *Epidemiologic Reviews, 29*(1), 6–28. doi:10.1093/epirev/mxm007.

Wang, A., Kinsinger, L., Kahwati, L., Das, S., Gizlice, Z., Harvey, R., et al. (2005). Obesity and weight controls practices in 2000 among veterans using VA facilities. *Obesity Research, 13*, 1405–1411. doi:10.1038/oby.2005.170.

Whyman, M., Lemmon, M., & Teachman, J. (2011). Non-combat military service in the United States and its effects on depressive symptoms among men. *Social Science Research, 40*(2), 695–703. doi:10.1016/j.ssresearch.2010.12.007.

Wilmoth, J. M., & London, A. S. (Eds.). (2013). *Life-course perspectives on military service.* New York: Routledge.

Wilmoth, J. M., London, A. S., & Heflin, C. M. (2015). Economic well-being among older-adult households: Variation by veteran and disability status. *Journal of Gerontological Social Work, 58*, 399–419.

Wilmoth, J. M., London, A. S., & Parker, W. M. (2010). Military service and men's health trajectories in later life. *The Journals of Gerontology. Series B, Psychological Sciences and Social Sciences, 56*(6), 744–755. doi:10.1093/geronb/gbq072.

Wolf, D. A., Wing, C., & Lopoo, L. M. (2013). Methodological problems in determining the consequences of military service. In J. M. Wilmoth & A. S. London (Eds.), *Life-course perspectives on military service* (pp. 254–274). New York: Routledge.

Chapter 8
Linear Mixed-Effects and Latent Curve Models for Longitudinal Life Course Analyses

Paolo Ghisletta, Olivier Renaud, Nadège Jacot, and Delphine Courvoisier

Introduction

The core of life course or lifespan research consists in studying how individual trajectories are shaped and unfold over time, from conception to death (Baltes 1987). Two concepts are fundamental in this endeavor: stability and change. Indeed, while certain individual characteristics remain constant across one's lifespan (e.g., sex, ethnicity), others undergo profound change, to the point that they might mutate into other characteristics (e.g., health, cognitive capacities). Such changes need not be independent of each other. They may simply co-occur, in the sense that while they happen simultaneously, it is hard to infer causality mechanisms between them. They may also be intrinsically related, where one change process is a necessary antecedent of the other, which becomes the consequence.

The empirical study of lifespan development necessitates hence statistical models capable, at the very least, of (a) estimating constancy and change in information from a collection of observed measurements and (b) assessing degrees of

P. Ghisletta (✉) • N. Jacot
Faculty of Psychology and Educational Sciences, University of Geneva, Geneva, Switzerland

Distance Learning University Switzerland, Brig, Switzerland
e-mail: paolo.ghisletta@unige.ch; nadege.jacot@unige.ch

O. Renaud
Faculty of Psychology and Educational Sciences, University of Geneva, Geneva, Switzerland
e-mail: olivier.renaud@unige.ch

D. Courvoisier
Division of Clinical Epidemiology, University Hospitals of Geneva, Geneva, Switzerland

Swiss National Center of Competence for Research LIVES – Overcoming Vulnerability: Life Course Perspectives, University of Geneva, Geneva, Switzerland
e-mail: delphine.courvoisier@unige.ch

© The Author(s) 2015

C. Burton-Jeangros et al. (eds.), *A Life Course Perspective on Health Trajectories and Transitions*, Life Course Research and Social Policies 4,
DOI 10.1007/978-3-319-20484-0_8

interrelationships among constant and changing characteristics. Moreover, in a contextual paradigm typical of life course research, it is also highly desirable to ascertain which characteristics are intrinsic to the individual and which are influenced by, or stem from, external factors. Thus, the statistical models adopted in life course research face a number of challenging questions, which in turn can only be met with an appropriate data collection methodology.

The Rationale and Objectives of Longitudinal Research

There is common agreement that to study any changing phenomenon it is best to utilize longitudinal data, rather than cross-sectional data with only one time of measurement per individual. Baltes and Nesselroade (1979), in their seminal chapter, have defined the rationale of longitudinal research as "the study of phenomena in their time-related constancy and change" (p. 2). This conceptualization encompasses various types of methodologies applied across many disciplines, such as panel or wave designs, repeated measurement experiments, single-subject designs, and time series. The common feature of these designs is the presence of repeated observations on the same units of observation (usually individuals). For instance, the same individuals are assessed multiple times, necessarily at different time points, and the researcher's interest lies in assessing what is constant, what changes across the multiple measurements, and what may explain the changes.

Following this rationale, Baltes and Nesselroade (1979) have outlined five objectives of longitudinal research. We repeat them here because these objectives motivate the use of longitudinal research and thereby should be directly addressed by statistical models applied to longitudinal data. To clarify, we provide a working example. The five objectives are:

- Direct identification of *intraindividual change*. This objective aims at estimating change over (at least two) repeated assessments at the individual level, thereby identifying individual trajectories of change. The estimation of intraindividual change is at the very heart of longitudinal research and can only be approximated (usually unsatisfactorily) by analyzing single measurements of different individuals assessed at different time points. Cross-sectional data, thus, do not allow the exploration of this objective. A researcher interested, for instance, in assessing social inequalities in health trajectories across the lifespan (e.g., Cullati et al. 2014) will start out by assessing whether the health status of individuals changes across time. Individuals for whom intraindividual change is observed will not display flat trajectories.
- Direct identification of *interindividual differences* (or similarities) *in intraindividual change*. In life course and lifespan research it is unrealistic to assume that entities are perfect replicates of each other. Hence, once intraindividual change is identified, this objective focuses on assessing whether individuals are similar

to or differ from each other with respect to their specific intraindividual change patterns. Indeed, while all individuals may change in time, some may display increase in the intensity of the observed behavior in time, while others may show decrease. To continue the previous example, it may well be that for some individuals their health trajectories are rather stable in time, while for others their trajectories decline, evincing deterioration in general health, or rise, signifying health improvement. Lack of interindividual differences in intraindividual change would be reflected by parallel health trajectories, meaning that all individuals' health changes equally.

- Analysis of *interrelationships in change*. It is seldom that life course researchers focus on single variables, because rarely do important characteristics of our lifespan change in a completely independent and autonomous fashion. Most often the interest lies in understanding how multiple variables are associated, either occurring in parallel, or influencing each other. For instance, change in one observed behavior (e.g., declining health) may occur in parallel with other characteristics (e.g., aging, socioeconomic status, increase in body mass index, loss of income), or be more likely to come about if another behavior is previously triggered (e.g., loss of employment). Such interrelationships, again, cannot be approximated by cross-sectional methodology, unless the characteristics are inert and do not undergo any change. That is, static correlations between cross-sectional assessments of behaviors are usually bad approximations of the dynamics at play between these behaviors.
- Analyses of *causes* (determinants) *of intraindividual change*. If intraindividual change can be identified (cf., first objective), it becomes highly pertinent to determine possible causes (or determinants) of such change. The passing of time is a convenient metric along which to describe and analyze change, but it seldom constitutes a theoretically sound explanation of any change process. While we know that in old age health generally declines, it is recognized that various causes are at play at very different levels (e.g., cellular, biological, epigenetic, psychological, social, all of which may correlate with aging).
- Analyses of *causes* (determinants) *of interindividual differences in intraindividual change*. If interindividual differences in intraindividual change (second objective) are detected, we may wonder what causes such differences. It may well be that the causes of intraindividual change (fourth objective) are different across individuals (e.g., while an individual's health improvement may primarily be due to change in marital status, another individual's health improvement might be triggered by change in occupation status). This fifth objective seems promising with regard to addressing social inequalities in health trajectories across the lifespan.

The statistical models we discuss in this chapter are widely used in many disciplines because they define parameters that address directly the five objectives of longitudinal research. Moreover, recent extensions of these models allow broadening the scopes of longitudinal research by exploring additional questions, such as the presence of interindividual differences due to (known or unknown) group membership. These models have also been adapted to handle realities of longitudinal designs which render the whole research enterprise more arduous, such as dealing with unavoidable missing values.

A Linear Model of Change

Let Y_{ij} represent the measurement of Y at time i for individual j. Let's assume there are $j = 1,2,\ldots,n$ individuals composing a sample of size n and let's assume this sample has been assessed at times $i = 1,2,\ldots T$, hence T times. The usual statistical assumption of such a sample is that the n individuals are independent of each other, meaning that the scores Y_{ij} of an individual j are not related to the scores $Y_{ij'}$ of another individual j', and this at any time point i. Nevertheless, it is natural to expect that the score Y_{ij} of individual j at time i is correlated with the score $Y_{i'j}$ of that same individual at another time point i', given that both depend on that individual's characteristics. The first objective of longitudinal research motivates understanding how the repeated measurements Y_{ij} are related in time. In other words, a mathematical model is wished for, to relate a meaningful variable that changes in time (hence assessed at multiple time points i) to the outcome of interest Y, and this for every individual j.

Historically, longitudinal data were first analyzed one individual at a time, separately, in what was named individual growth models (the term growth most probably is due to the fact that the first applications of this kind studied the physical growth of children undergoing puberty; see McArdle 2001). In other words, for n individuals, n models were computed separately. In this context, most frequently the repeated assessments were related to the aging of the individual, where a_{ij} is the age of individual j at time i. Note that other definitions of time can be specified (e.g., occasions of measurement, assessment trials in a laboratory experiment, hours of the day when studying a circadian function). A simple model assuming that Y is linearly related to age (a_{ij}) is the simple linear regression model as specified in Eq. 8.1. Because this model has to be estimated separately for each individual j, we drop the subscript j.

$$Y_i = \pi_0 + \pi_1 a_i + E_i \qquad (8.1)$$

In the end, the analyst will obtain, for each individual j, a value for: (a) the intercept π_0, which defines the predicted value of Y when age $= 0$; (b) the slope π_1, which defines the predicted change (either positive for growth or negative for decline) of Y for each unit change (e.g., one year, one month) in age; (c) the standard error of the estimate, which is closely related to the variability of the errors E_i at each time point and which defines the quality of the overall age prediction of Y. Note that to interpret the intercept, it is customary to center age around a meaningful value, such as the average of the sample (by subtracting from each individual's age the sample average age). The intercept is then the predicted Y value for an individual of average age. Alternative age scalings have been proposed and might allow for a more meaningful interpretation of the intercept in particular research situations (e.g., Mehta and West 2000; Wainer 2000). The assumptions of the model are that the errors E_i are normally distributed (i.e., they follow a normal, Gaussian curve) and do not depend on values of age (i.e., homoscedasticity).

If the model is estimated for each individual, n estimates of these parameters are obtained. Of course, other mathematical relations between age and Y can be tested, such as polynomial or exponential functions (for instance, to model human growth, various exponential functions have been proposed). What must be kept in mind is that so far the analysis is individual-specific. At the first analytical step, the growth model is estimated for each individual. At the second analytical step, the individual estimates are subsequently summarized. Any conclusion about the overall sample would have to be inferred by summarizing the n estimates, for instance by calculating the average and the variance of the intercepts and of the slopes across all individuals. Note that the two steps are computed independently of each other.

The Linear Mixed-Effects Model

In 1982 Laird and Ware proposed a model that allowed estimating simultaneously intercept and slope information at both the individual and the sample level. The model is an expansion of the individual growth model and is presented in Eq. 8.2.

$$Y_{ij} = \pi_{0j} + \pi_{1j}a_{ij} + E_{ij}$$
$$\pi_{0j} = \beta_0 + U_{0j} \tag{8.2}$$
$$\pi_{1j} = \beta_1 + U_{1j}$$

Given that the repeated assessments of Y of all individuals are analyzed simultaneously, Eq. 8.2 necessitates the addition of the subscript j, which identifies the individual. Moreover, this approach supposes one set of growth parameters, that is, one intercept and one slope, per individual, which again justifies the subscript j on both parameters π_0 and π_1. Technically, it is not correct to say that an intercept and a slope value are estimated for each individual. That is, the model does not explicitly estimate a π_{0j} and a π_{1j} value for each individual j. The model presupposes, however, that each individual may have an intercept and a slope value that deviate from the central (population average) values, which are indicated by β_0 and β_1 and which are explicitly estimated. What are also estimated are the inter-individual variances, due to the individual deviations U_{0j} and U_{1j} around the central values, and possibly the covariance between U_{0j} and U_{1j}. The variances of the U_{0j} and U_{1j} are defined by the parameters σ^2_I and σ^2_S, respectively, and their covariance by the parameter σ_{IS}. Lastly, the errors of prediction E_{ij} are not individually estimated. These are often assumed to have a constant variance in time, estimated by the parameter σ^2_E, and to be uncorrelated in time. In sum, then, in its

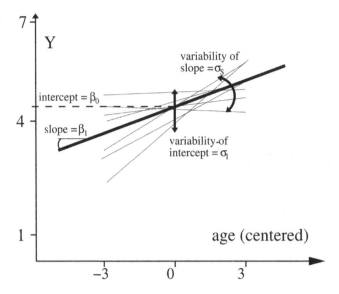

Fig. 8.1 Schematic representation of the parameters estimated in the LMEM (Eq. 8.2). The thin lines represent the best-fitting trajectory of each individual, while the thick line represents the best-fitting trajectory based on the central values (representative of the overall sample). In this example the value of the slope, β_1, is positive. Note that the estimated slope variance, $\sigma^2{}_S$, and intercept-slope covariance, σ_{IS}, depend on where age has been centered

most frequent specification, this model estimates six parameters: two central values, for the intercept, β_0, and the slope, β_1, two variances and a covariance of growth parameters, $\sigma^2{}_I$, $\sigma^2{}_S$, and σ_{IS}, and an error variance $\sigma^2{}_E$. Figure 8.1 illustrates schematically the parameters of the *linear mixed-effects model* (LMEM).

This model distinguishes two kinds of parameters: the central values, which are common to all individuals (β_0 and β_1) and are called *fixed effects*, and the individual deviations from these central values (U_{0j} and U_{1j}), called the *random effects*. Again, the random effects and the individual errors (E_{ij}) are not directly estimated, but their variances and covariance ($\sigma^2{}_I$, $\sigma^2{}_S$, σ_{IS}, and $\sigma^2{}_E$) are. Fixed effects thus apply to all individuals and are not subject to individual variations. Random effects, on the other hand, vary across individuals and do so by typically following the standard distribution of random variables, that is, a normal (Gaussian) distribution. The model hence assumes that all random effects (U_{0j}, U_{1j}) and errors (E_{ij}) are normally distributed (symbolized by $U_{0j} \sim \mathcal{N}(0, \sigma^2{}_I)$, $U_{1j} \sim \mathcal{N}(0, \sigma^2{}_S)$, and $E_{ij} \sim \mathcal{N}(0, \sigma^2{}_E)$), that the random effects may covary ($\mathrm{Cov}(U_{0j}, U_{1j}) = \sigma_{IS}$), that the errors do not covary with the random effects ($\mathrm{Cov}(E_{ij}, U_{0j}) = \mathrm{Cov}(E_{ij}, U_{1j}) = 0$), and that the errors do not covary in time ($\mathrm{Cov}(E_{ij}, E_{i'j}) = 0$).

The coexistence of fixed and random effects within the same model gives it the name of the linear mixed-effects model. The term linear denotes that the function linking Y to the predictor a_{ij} is linear in its parameters, meaning that the parameters associated to the prediction of Y (on the right side of the equal sign in Eq. 8.2) are at most multiplied by a predictor and then added (i.e., the prediction is a linear combination of the parameters and the predictors), rather than, for instance, being exponentiated. This model has been developed in different disciplines, and is also known as random-effects model (Laird and Ware 1982), hierarchical linear model (Bryk and Raudenbush 1987), and multilevel model (Goldstein 1989).

The LMEM of Eq. 8.2 has notable advantages over the individually estimated growth models of Eq. 8.1. First, the estimation is simultaneous, that is, instead of involving two analytical steps it can be computed in a single step. All n individuals' data are analyzed together, in a single analysis. This makes for a considerable gain in time. Second, the statistical tests obtained with the LMEM are superior to those of individually estimated growth models. More precisely, the Type I error rate of statistical tests is closer to its nominal value within the LMEM than in individual growth models, which are usually too liberal (Snijders and Bosker 2012). Third, the LMEM allows for a statistical test of sample heterogeneity, which is not possible with the individual growth approach. Hence, statistical tests for the significance of variances and covariance of the random effects (σ^2_I, σ^2_S, and σ_{IS}) are possible within the LMEM. This feature is extremely important, as these parameters represent heterogeneity in growth parameters, a concept often of chief interest from a theoretical perspective. Fourth, the LMEM can be extended to define parameters that operationalize the five objectives of longitudinal research: (a) Intraindividual change is directly identified with the first line of Eq. 8.2, and β_0 and β_1 define the average intraindividual change function; (b) the intercept variance σ^2_I and the slope variance σ^2_S identify directly interindividual differences in intraindividual change; (c) in multivariate specifications of the LMEM it is possible to covary intercept and slope of one change process with those of another (MacCallum et al. 1997; more detail in the section "Three Notable Extensions", below); (d) it is straightforward to add a predictor to the first line of Eq. 8.2 to test a determinant of intraindividual change; and (e) if intercept variance and slope variance are significant, it is straightforward to extend the LMEM to include a predictor of interindividual differences in intraindividual change (more detail in the section "Inclusion of Covariates", below). In other words, the LMEM appears to provide explicit statistical tests directly associated to the rationale and objectives of longitudinal research enunciated by Baltes and Nesselroade (1979). Consequently, this statistical model addresses key theoretical questions of life course research.

The Latent Curve Model

In 1984, Meredith and Tisak 1984 presented the precepts of how the LMEM defined above can be specified as a structural equation model. The work was later formalized by the same authors (Meredith and Tisak 1990), and applied by McArdle (1986). Structural equation modeling can largely be defined as a set of statistical techniques aimed at testing hypothesized relationships among chosen variables. In this context, the Latent Curve Model (LCM) formalizes how a series of repeated measurements of variable Y for individual j, represented by the vector $\mathbf{Y_j}$, is related to the passing of time (or aging of the individual) as specified in Eq. 8.3 (note that it is customary to write the names of vectors and matrices in boldface).

$$\mathbf{Y_j} = \Lambda\boldsymbol{\eta}_j + \mathbf{E_j} \tag{8.3}$$

For each individual j, the T repeated measurements of Y are piled up in the vector $\mathbf{Y_j}$ (of size $T \times 1$, corresponding to Y_{1j} to Y_{Tj} in Eq. 8.2). $\boldsymbol{\eta}_j$ represents the vector (of size 2×1) of the two growth factors (or latent variables), intercept and slope (equivalent to π_{0j} and π_{1j} in Eq. 8.2). Λ is the matrix (of size $T \times 2$) of the factor loadings associating the repeated observations to the growth factors. Note that Λ is not indexed by j, indicating that its values are the same for all individuals. Finally, $\mathbf{E_j}$ is the vector (of size $T \times 1$, corresponding to E_{1j} up to E_{Tj} in Eq. 8.2) of time-specific errors. The loadings associating the intercept to the measurements (i.e., the first column of Λ) are conveniently fixed at 1 (the multiplier of π_{0j} in Eq. 8.2). To specify linear change, the loadings of the slope factor (i.e., the second column of Λ) increase linearly with time, or age. Hence, in this basic specification, the elements of the loading matrix Λ are not estimated. For instance, if the sample is observed at five ages, the loadings of the intercept would be $[1\ 1\ 1\ 1\ 1]'$ while for the slope they might be $[-2\ -1\ 0\ 1\ 2]'$, (the values of a_{ij} in Eq. 8.2; the prime symbol ' stands for transposed). This is equivalent to centering the variable age on the third value in the LMEM. To clarify, we expand the general LCM notation in an illustration below (cf. Eq. 8.7).

The crucial parameter estimates of the LCM are associated to the growth factors $\boldsymbol{\eta}$. The central values of the intercept and of the slope factor correspond to the fixed effects β_0 and β_1 of the LMEM; the variances of the two factors correspond to σ^2_I and σ^2_S and their covariance corresponds to σ_{IS}. Finally, if the error variance is constrained to be constant in time, its estimate corresponds to σ^2_E. In the end, it can be shown that, while they have originated in rather widely different fields of statistics, the LMEM and the LCM as specified here are completely equivalent (e.g., Bauer 2003; Chou et al. 1998; McArdle and Hamagami 1996).

Inclusion of Covariates

The growth model implemented via the LMEM or the LCM allows for testing sample heterogeneity in the growth factors. For instance, are individuals different from each other with respect to their intercept score? This question is operational-ized by testing the null hypothesis that the intercept variance is zero (H_0: $\sigma^2_I = 0$). Likewise, we can ask whether there are individual differences in the change process, or whether the entities are different from each other with respect to their slope score. Testing the null hypothesis of zero slope variance (H_0: $\sigma^2_S = 0$) addresses this question. If there appear to be interindividual differences in intercept and in slope (i.e., if the two variances are different from zero), a natural question is whether the intercept and the slope scores are related. This question is addressed by the null hypothesis of zero covariance (H_0: $\sigma_{IS} = 0$).

If sample heterogeneity in intercept and/or slope appears significant, we can wonder whether a given characteristic of the entity may influence the growth factors. This question can easily be addressed within the LMEM and LCM by expanding the models to include predictors. There are two kinds of predictors. Time-varying predictors are those that vary across time, such as a medical or physical measurement taken at each assessment time, and hence require not only a subscript j to determine the individual, but also a subscript i to specify their time of assessment. These predictors are also called time-dependent or level 1 and may help explain intraindividual change. Time-invariant predictors, on the other hand, are individual specific and do not change in time, such as sex. These are simply denoted with a subscript j and are also called level 2, and may help explain interindividual differences in intraindividual change.

The LMEM can be expanded to include a time-varying predictor x_{ij} and a time-invariant predictor z_j as shown in Eq. 8.4.

$$
\begin{aligned}
Y_{ij} &= \pi_{0j} + \pi_{1j}a_{ij} + \pi_2 x_{ij} + E_{ij} \\
\pi_{0j} &= \beta_{00} + \beta_{01}z_j + U_{0j} \\
\pi_{1j} &= \beta_{10} + \beta_{11}z_j + U_{1j}
\end{aligned}
\tag{8.4}
$$

In the LCM the inclusion of a time-varying and a time-invariant predictor is shown in Eq. 8.5 (in which we use the notation that is standard in the structural equation modeling literature; e.g., Bollen and Curran 2006).

$$
\begin{aligned}
\mathbf{Y}_j &= \Lambda \boldsymbol{\eta}_j + B\mathbf{x}_j + \mathbf{E}_j \\
\boldsymbol{\eta}_j &= \boldsymbol{\alpha} + \boldsymbol{\Gamma}\boldsymbol{\xi}_j + \boldsymbol{\zeta}_j
\end{aligned}
\tag{8.5}
$$

Equation 8.5 specifies that the outcome $\mathbf{Y}_j$ is not only influenced by the growth factors $\boldsymbol{\eta}_j$, but also by an observed time-varying covariate $\mathbf{x}_j$, through a regression weight specified in the scalar B (equivalent to π_2 in Eq. 8.4). The vector $\mathbf{x}_j$ has T rows and one column, while the scalar B is a single number. The growth factors $\boldsymbol{\eta}_j$ may be influenced by a time-invariant covariate ξ_j (z_j in Eq. 8.4) via the regression intercepts $\boldsymbol{\alpha}$ (β_{00} and β_{10} in Eq. 8.4) and the regression weights $\boldsymbol{\Gamma}$ (β_{01} and β_{11} in Eq. 8.4). Given that the prediction of $\boldsymbol{\eta}_j$ by ξ_j will likely not be perfect in practice, Eq. 8.5 includes the regression errors $\boldsymbol{\zeta}_j$ (U_{0j} and U_{1j} in Eq. 8.4). Again, it can be shown that the models in Eqs. 8.4 and 8.5 are equivalent.

Note that it is not necessary that a time-invariant predictor influence both the intercept and the slope. Just like in ordinary linear regression, multiple predictors, including interactions, can be added to the model. Also, the same substantive variable could be considered as time-varying (for instance, daily values of a characteristic) or as time-invariant (for example, average value of the same characteristic over multiple days). In such cases it is important to note that the meaning of the variable can change dramatically and special care must be taken when interpreting the results (Goldstein 2011; Raudenbush and Bryk 2002; Snijders and Bosker 2012). Also, the LCM allows for more flexibility when testing covariates' effects. For instance, the effect of a time-varying predictor is typically specified to be the same at all time points in the LMEM. While relaxing this equality constraint requires some data manipulation in LMEM, this can easily be achieved in the LCM.

We expect the variability of the random effects and of the errors (i.e., σ^2_I, σ^2_S, and σ^2_E) to diminish as we add important predictors to the model. In other words, the unexplained variance of the models should decrease as we add important predictors (this effect can be tested statistically). Effect size measures, similar to the coefficient of determination (R^2) in ordinary linear regression, have been proposed to quantify these effects (e.g., Snijders and Bosker 1994).

LMEM or LCM?

Given the equivalency of the two models, when should an analyst use the LMEM and when the LCM? To a certain extent, the answer is a matter of preference. Given that the two approaches stem from different traditions, historically the statistical programs estimating these models were quite specific. Either they would estimate the LMEM (e.g., MIXED in SPSS, PROC MIXED in SAS, nlme and lme4 in R, mixed in STATA, HLM, MLwiN) or the LCM (e.g., LiSRel, AMOS, Mx, OpenMx in R, sem in STATA, EQS, Mplus). Recently, some software allow for both estimations (e.g., R, LiSRel, Mplus), although the optimization algorithms implemented in such software may not be the most efficient.

There are, however, empirical conditions, in which the implementation of one model over the other may be indicated. Ghisletta and Lindenberger (2004) described the relative advantages and disadvantages of the LMEM and the LCM approaches and suggested some practical guidelines concerning the choice between the two. In brief, the LMEM may be preferable over the LCM when (a) the data set is not balanced (i.e., not every entity has been observed at all times and at the same time points; hence, each entity j has been observed T_j times, where T_j may vary across entities) and there are many incomplete data; (b) the theoretical functional form of change is a common mathematical function (e.g., linear, polynomial, exponential); (c) the structure of the error covariance matrix is common (e.g., independent-diagonal, auto-regressive, unstructured); (d) the theoretical relation between the growth factors (i.e., intercept and slope) can only be a covariance (rather than, for instance, a regression weight); and (e) the role of a time-invariant variable, characteristic of the individual (e.g., sex, ethnicity, age at study inception), is that of predicting the growth factors, rather than for instance correlating with them.

The LCM approach may be more indicated than the LMEM approach when (a) there is a limited amount of unbalanced and incomplete data; (b) the change function is more complex than common mathematical functions (but remains linear in its parameters) or, when unknown, may be estimated directly from the data; (c) the structure of the errors is of theoretical interest and requires flexible specifications; (d) the growth factors are not limited to simply covary but could be regressed on each other; and (e) the associations between external covariates and the growth factors are not limited to unilateral predictions.

These suggestions are meant as starting guidelines and not definite rules. Either approach has undergone notable extensions, which greatly amplifies their degree of flexibility in modeling change processes. For instance, the LMEM has been extended to allow relating the outcome (Y_{ij}) to the predictors (on the right side of Eqs. 8.2 or 8.4) by a so-called link function from the exponential family. This model is called the Generalized Linear Mixed Model (GLMM; McCulloch and Searle 2001). Even more flexibility about the relationships between the outcome and the predictors has been introduced in the context of the so-called Nonlinear Mixed-Effects Models (Davidian and Giltinan 1995). The LCM has also undergone notable extensions. In particular, when applied to multiple variables, the model has been extended to include dynamic associations between the growth factors, allowing to establish which variable, if any, is driving the change of the other variable, hence determining the leader and the lagger within a multivariate dynamic system (McArdle and Hamagami 2001).

An Illustration from the Swiss Household Panel

To illustrate the LMEM and the LCM, we use data from the second sample of the Swiss Household Panel (SHP), which is a study based at the Swiss Centre of Expertise in the Social Sciences FORS. The project is financed by the Swiss National Science Foundation. The SHP is a nationally representative survey of households investigating trends in social dynamics among the Swiss population. Data are collected annually by Computer Assisted Telephone Interviewing. For this illustration, we focus on eight waves collected on 3,665 individuals, running from 2004 to 2011, and examine the evolution of self-reported health (SRH) over time. SRH is measured by the first question of the Short-Form-36 ("In general, do you think your health is...", rated from 1 (excellent) to 5 (poor)). Albeit simple, this measure is interesting because it predicts several important health outcomes, such as sick leave, and mortality (Berkman and Syme 1979; Halford et al. 2012).

We reverse coded SRH, such that 1 represents poor health and 5 indicates excellent health. Independent variables are sex (sex_j, coded 0 for men and 1 for women), a time-invariant predictor, and satisfaction with personal relationships ($satrel_{ij}$, rated from 0, not at all satisfied, to 10, completely satisfied), a time-varying predictor. In addition, to examine intraindividual change in SRH and allow for the influence of sex on this change, we included time ($time_{ij}$) as a time-varying predictor, yielding the following model:

LMEM Notation

$$SRH_{ij} = \pi_{0j} + \pi_{1j}time_{ij} + \pi_2 satrel_{ij} + E_{ij}$$
$$\pi_{0j} = \beta_{00} + \beta_{01}sex_j + U_{0j} \tag{8.6}$$
$$\pi_{1j} = \beta_{10} + \beta_{11}sex_j + U_{1j}$$

LCM Notation

$$
\begin{pmatrix} SRH_{1j} \\ SRH_{2j} \\ SRH_{3j} \\ SRH_{4j} \\ SRH_{5j} \\ SRH_{6j} \\ SRH_{7j} \\ SRH_{8j} \end{pmatrix} = \begin{pmatrix} 1 & 0 \\ 1 & 1 \\ 1 & 2 \\ 1 & 3 \\ 1 & 4 \\ 1 & 5 \\ 1 & 6 \\ 1 & 7 \end{pmatrix} \begin{pmatrix} \eta_{1j} \\ \eta_{2j} \end{pmatrix} + B \begin{pmatrix} satrel_{1j} \\ satrel_{2j} \\ satrel_{3j} \\ satrel_{4j} \\ satrel_{5j} \\ satrel_{6j} \\ satrel_{7j} \\ satrel_{8j} \end{pmatrix} + \begin{pmatrix} E_{1j} \\ E_{2j} \\ E_{3j} \\ E_{4j} \\ E_{5j} \\ E_{6j} \\ E_{7j} \\ E_{8j} \end{pmatrix} \tag{8.7}
$$

$$
\begin{pmatrix} \eta_{1j} \\ \eta_{2j} \end{pmatrix} = \begin{pmatrix} \alpha_1 \\ \alpha_2 \end{pmatrix} + \begin{pmatrix} \Gamma_1 \\ \Gamma_2 \end{pmatrix} sex_j + \begin{pmatrix} \zeta_{1j} \\ \zeta_{2j} \end{pmatrix}
$$

We used the `lme4` and `OpenMx` packages in the R environment (R Core Team 2013) to estimate the models (for the code: see Appendix). Results are shown in Table 8.1 (all estimates are significant at the $\alpha = 1\%$ level, unless otherwise indicated). We can see that SRH decreases slightly over time (β_{10} in LMEM notation, cf. Eq. 8.6; α_1 in LCM notation, cf. Eq. 8.7), and that women report slightly poorer health (β_{01}; Γ_1). Furthermore, women and men have similar overall intraindividual change in SRH (β_{11}; Γ_2 are non-significant). Satisfaction with personal relationships has a positive association with SRH (π_2; B), so that an increase of 1 point in satisfaction with relationships yields a 0.044 (0.043 in the LCM) increase in SRH. Finally, compared to the error variance (σ^2_E), there is a relatively large interindividual variability in SRH (σ^2_I), and a small variability in intraindividual change (σ^2_S). The covariance between the random intercept and random slope (correlation $= -0.38$) indicates that individuals with higher initial SRH have a tendency to decline faster (a larger negative slope) than individuals with lower SRH.

As can be seen from the results displayed in Table 8.1, the solutions estimated from the LMEM and LCM are virtually identical. The slight differences are not meaningful and can be imputed to differences in the optimization algorithms adopted by the two approaches.

Table 8.1 Estimates of LMEM and LCM to predict evolution of SRH over time with sex and satisfaction with relationships as independent variables

Independent variables	LMEM		LCM	
	Notation	Estimate	Notation	Estimate
Intercept	β_{00}	3.760	α_1	3.760
Sex (ref: male)	β_{01}	−0.135	Γ_1	−0.133
Time (for males)	β_{10}	−0.015	α_2	−0.015
Interaction time: sex	β_{11}	0.001^{ns}	Γ_2	0.0004^{ns}
Satisfaction with relationships	π_2	0.044	B	0.043
Intercept variance	σ^2_I	0.223	σ^2_I	0.227
Slope variance	σ^2_S	0.002	σ^2_S	0.002
Covariance intercept-slope	σ_{IS}	−0.009	σ_{IS}	−0.009
Error variance	σ^2_E	0.252	σ^2_E	0.253

Source of data: Swiss Household Panel
ns non-significant at $\alpha = 1\%$

Three Notable Extensions

Both the LMEM and the LCM have been extended to accommodate three notable features. First, because of the practical realities of any longitudinal study, a statistical model aimed at analyzing longitudinal data must be able to handle incomplete data. For instance, in any long-term longitudinal study lasting several weeks, months, years, or decades it is virtually impossible that all participants present at inception remain for the total duration. So-called micro-longitudinal studies (such as a psychological experiments lasting a few minutes, during which individuals are repeatedly assessed) are not necessarily immune to this type of dropout mechanism, either. This gives rise to data being incomplete for some, often most, participants.

Pretending data to be complete by limiting one's analyses to the entities that provided all longitudinal assessments (so-called complete-case analyses) will most likely lead to biased estimation, because the subsample with complete data usually represents a selection of the starting sample. That is, the parameter estimates obtained from the application of any statistical model to complete-case longitudinal data will likely be different (biased) from the population parameters. Note that it is not the quantity of data incompleteness that is necessarily the chief determinant of the amount of estimation bias, but rather the nature of (the process causing) incomplete data.

Second, the frequent use of the LMEM and LCM to single variables assessed repeatedly has motivated multivariate applications to address relations in change processes. It is not realistic, for any substantive life course researcher, to theorize single behaviors or attitudes in isolation. Most often, from a theoretical perspective, it is most interesting to study interrelationships between multiple variables, to assess, for instance, if an entity changing on one behavior also tends to change on another behavior. Multivariate extensions of both the LMEM and the LCM easily address such questions.

Third, it is often illusory to assume that the samples at hand represent homogeneous groupings of entities. We may have reasons to believe that known characteristics of the entities may influence their change process. Males vs. females, wealthy vs. poor, with a low vs. a high level of education, etc. may differ from each other. Rather than considering such characteristics as covariates in the LMEM and LCM, it is possible to use them to create subsamples, which are then compared with respect to all parameters of the models. Moreover, group membership may not be known, but uncovered, in a rather exploratory fashion, from the data. This last application has received wide attention in several disciplines studying the life course.

Incomplete Data

Virtually every longitudinal study faces the reality of not having all assessments at all time points on all participants. For instance, in the illustration above, by the end of the study 50.4% of the initial participants were no longer in the study. Modern methods allow obtaining unbiased estimates despite the incompleteness of the outcome data Y. Under specific conditions (see Rubin 1976), any variable X that may be related to the reasons of data incompleteness in Y is called informative or auxiliary. For instance, older and less healthy participants are more likely to drop out of a longitudinal study than younger and healthier participants. Thus, age and health are informative X variables that are related to the probability of not providing outcome Y values. Informative variables can be added to a longitudinal model to decrease estimation bias. This is why it is of chief importance to measure as many potentially informative X variables as possible at the first wave of a longitudinal study, when attrition (i.e., incomplete data in Y) has not yet occurred. This information may be used in subsequent waves to lessen estimation bias (for more detail, see Graham 2009, and Schafer and Graham 2002). In the previous illustration, satisfaction with personal relationships was related to the probability of dropping out, so that its inclusion in the model does not only address an interesting substantive issue but also reduces overall estimation bias.

In some situations it is desirable to have incomplete data, mainly to avoid other, more deleterious effects. For instance, to understand the interrelationships among a very big set of variables, it is not necessary to administer all variables to all participants. Doing so could introduce major fatigue and demotivation effects, which are likely to lower the validity and reliability of the assessments. Rather, it is possible to randomly create subgroups of participants, each of which is administered a reduced set of variables. What matters is that the subsets of variables overlap across the participants, so that all interrelationships among the variables can be estimated. If carefully planned, then, the administration time and participants' burden can be reduced dramatically, without increase in parameter bias nor the need for informative variables (McArdle 1994).

In longitudinal research this feature may be of crucial importance. Researchers interested in wide segments of the life course (say, young adulthood, from age

18 to 35 years) can probably not afford to observe an age-homogeneous sample during the entire time epoch of interest (that is, study a sample of 18-year old participants during 17 years, until they are 35 years old). By the means of so-called age-convergence analyses (Bell 1953, 1954) and cohort sequential designs (Schaie 1977), it is possible to reduce the overall length of the study, without having to shorten the time epoch of substantive interest. For instance, three samples, of 18-, 23-, and 28-year old participants, may be observed for seven years. The total interval of time is now covered in seven rather than 17 years, and the partial age overlap of the three samples (18–25, 23–30, and 28–35 years) will allow testing whether the samples develop alike (i.e., convergence).

The software implementing the LMEM is more flexible than that of LCM analyses when dealing with incomplete Y data. Indeed, the optimization algorithms used to estimate parameters with incomplete data sets are usually much more efficient for the LMEM. Nevertheless, the LCM allows for a more flexible treatment of informative covariates, so that in problematic instances of incomplete data the LCM may be the preferred strategy (Graham 2003). However, neither the LMEM nor the LCM compensate directly for missing X values. In that case, two valuable alternative strategies are to either apply multiple imputation first, to impute all incomplete X and Y values, and then apply the longitudinal model (e.g., Carpenter and Goldstein 2004), or to estimate the model in the Bayesian framework (e.g., Muthén and Muthén 1998–2012).

Multivariate Extensions

By definition, a statistical model for longitudinal data must involve multiple variables, in that the outcome of interest must be observed at least twice (at times $i = 1$ and $i = 2$). Despite this technicality, it is common to call a longitudinal model applied to a single outcome *univariate*, denoting that a single Y outcome is analyzed. It follows that a *multivariate* longitudinal model is one that analyzes at least two outcomes (Y_1 and Y_2). In its simplest specification, a multivariate LMEM supposes an intercept and a slope growth factor for each outcome, which covary freely (MacCallum et al. 1997). This allows assessing the degree of communality of multiple change processes. Note that the functional form of growth need not be the same across the outcomes. In the previous illustration it would be possible to study change in both self-rated health and satisfaction with personal relationships. A multivariate LMEM might specify an intercept and a slope for both outcomes and estimate all six covariances among the four growth factors.

The LCM can also be easily adapted to multiple outcomes. Here, the association between the growth factors is not limited to symmetrical effects (i.e., covariances), but may be freely specified by the analyst. For instance, it is possible to let the growth factors of an earlier process predict those of a later process (rather than simply covary with them; Singer and Willett 2003). Such a relation cannot be tested within a multivariate LMEM. In the previous illustration we might want to assess the effect of degree of satisfaction with personal relationship and change therein on self-rated health. Then, we might define a multivariate LCM with satisfaction assessments from 2004 to 2007 and health assessments from 2008 to 2011. We could then estimate the effects of the intercept and slope of the former (and temporally preceding) construct on the intercept and slope of the latter.

Another important multivariate extension of the LCM stems from its implementation within the structural equation modeling framework, where it is possible to define latent variables based on the common, shared variance of a chosen set of observed variables via a common factor model (Spearman 1904). Assuming the common factor can be defined at each wave of measurement of a longitudinal study, the outcome of interest is no longer an observed variable, but the latent variable itself. A LCM (with growth factors of higher order) can hence be specified to assess the growth of the common factor (McArdle called this extension a Curve of Factors Model; McArdle 1988). For instance, rather than relying on a single health question, multiple questions (and/or objective health measurements) could be assessed, to define a common health factor. The LCM would then study the change trajectory not of the single health assessments, but of the common health factor.

Specific multivariate extensions of the LMEM/LCM are particularly useful when trying to assess causality relations between multiple outcomes. For instance, the LCM can be modified to define multiple slope factors, each acting between two adjacent i-1 and i assessments. Then, each assessment at time i-1 can influence the immediately upcoming change between i-1 and i. In a bivariate setting it is then possible to estimate, for instance, the influence of variable A at time i-1 on the change in variable B between i-1 and i, and vice-versa. This analysis would allow determining whether satisfaction with personal relationships drives changes in self-assessed health, or vice-versa, or both variables influence each other's change. Similar extensions are possible within the multivariate LMEM, with the inclusion of instrumental variables to predict time-invariant and/or time-varying confounders (e.g., Skrondal and Rabe-Hesketh 2004). However, for this extension, as well as for all models discussed here, it is important to bear in mind that they cannot be considered as proofs of causal relationships, because it is not conceivable to assure that no other construct or variable is causing such relationships.

Multiple Group Analyses

The specifications of growth models discussed thus far assume that the sample is homogeneous with respect to the growth process, meaning that all entities within the sample follow the same functional form of growth (albeit allowing for interindividual differences with respect to the magnitude of the growth factors – i.e., random effects). Adding a time-invariant covariate that clearly splits the overall sample in subsamples (e.g., men and women), as discussed in Eqs. 8.4 and 8.5, allows for a difference in mean intercept and mean slope between men and women. However, all other parameters and the shape of change remain unaltered across the sexes. The adequacy of this constraint can be tested. A multiple-group analysis, by sex, of the previous illustration would reveal that men and women have different mean intercepts of health (with women's inferior to men's), but similar mean slopes (consistent with the non-significant time-by-sex interaction in Table 8.1).

Splitting the sample into two subsamples allows freeing the equality constraints of all remaining parameters, as well as recovering group-specific growth features that would otherwise go unobserved. For instance, in a clinical trial we would expect a treatment group to react differently from a control group, not just with respect to the average intercept and slope mean, but much more generally. The control group may not undergo any change and remain constant. Hence, the growth model may be reduced to an intercept-only model. The treatment group would probably undergo marked change, as a result of the treatment, which would require the growth model to specify factors to this effect. Such a group difference cannot be modeled by considering group membership as a simple covariate.

In yet other cases we may suspect the existence of different subgroups, with respect to the analyzed change process, but ignore both the groups' characteristics and individual group membership. Thus, in a standard LCM, we cannot split the sample into subsamples according to the values of a known grouping variable. In this case, the grouping variable is assumed latent or unobserved, and we ignore its values. Recent developments extended the LCM to allow uncovering subgroups based on latent grouping variables. Latent class growth analyses (Nagin 1999) and growth mixture models (Muthén et al. 2002) are two such models, and both are currently only implemented in the LCM framework. Advanced versions of this approach can also be applied to state-trait type models, in order to uncover groups of individuals based on their degree of variability vs. stability (Courvoisier et al. 2007).

Conclusions

The LMEM and the LCM are statistical models of change that have permeated in many scientific disciplines. Today, they are largely used, thanks also to excellent reviews and textbooks, often supplemented by online material (e.g., Collins 2006; Duncan et al. 2006; McArdle and Nesselroade 2014; Pinheiro and Bates 2000; Singer and Willett 2003). Additionally, university curricula in psychology, sociology, demography, gerontology, and other disciplines related to the study of the life course have started integrating courses or workshops that discuss, among other statistical models, the LMEM and the LCM.

We believe that disciplines concerned with the study of the life course and the lifespan can greatly benefit from using the LMEM and the LCM. At the same time, we do not conceive statistics to be an independent academic discipline that mainly provides tools to substantive researchers. The many theoretical and methodological challenges of life course research call for flexible statistical tools. Ideally, statisticians and substantive life course researchers engage in dialogues and make progress together. Increased use of the LMEM and the LCM by life course researchers will motivate statisticians to additionally extend both models. With this chapter we hope to have further encouraged this dialogue.

Appendix

```
##################################################################
# Ghisletta, P., Renaud, O., Jacot, N., and Courvoisier, D. (2014)
# Linear mixed-effects and latent curve models for
# longitudinal life course analyses.
# In Burton-Jeangros, C., Cullati, S., and Sacker, A. (Eds).
# A life course perspective on health trajectories and transitions
# Berlin, Germany: Springer
#
#
#       R code for analyses on Swiss Household Panel, 2004-2011
#
#
##################################################################


# Import the data
shp.data <- read.table(file="shp04_11.csv",
                       header=TRUE, sep=";")

# Select the variables of interest
shp <- shp.data[,c("IDPERS", "SEX",
                   "P04C01", "P05C01",
                   "P06C01", "P07C01",
                   "P08C01", "P09C01",
                   "P10C01", "P11C01",
                   "P04QL04", "P05QL04",
                   "P06QL04", "P07QL04",
                   "P08QL04", "P09QL04",
                   "P10QL04", "P11QL04")]


######
# LMEM

###############################
# Reshape data in a long format
shp.lmem <- reshape(shp, idvar="IDPERS", times=0:7,
                    direction="long",
                    varying=list(c("P04C01", "P05C01",
                                   "P06C01", "P07C01",
                                   "P08C01", "P09C01",
                                   "P10C01", "P11C01"),
                                 c("P04QL04", "P05QL04",
                                   "P06QL04", "P07QL04",
                                   "P08QL04", "P09QL04",
                                   "P10QL04", "P11QL04")),
                    v.names=c("SRH", "SATREL"))

# Replace the values inferior to 1 by NA for the variable SRH
shp.lmem$SRH[shp.lmem$SRH<1] <- NA

# Replace the values inferior to 0 by NA for the variable SATREL
shp.lmem$SATREL[shp.lmem$SATREL<0] <- NA

# Load the package car that contains the function recode()
```

```
library(car)

# Recode the variable SRH in order to have
# 1=poor health and 5=excellent health
shp.lmem$SRH <- recode(shp.lmem$SRH, "1=5 ; 2=4; 3=3; 4=2; 5=1")

# Recode the variable sex in order to have 0=male and 1=female
shp.lmem$SEX <- shp.lmem$SEX-1

############
# Estimation

# Load the package lme4 that contains the function lmer()
library(lme4)

# Fit the model
LMEM.model <- lmer(SRH ~ 1+ SEX*time + SATREL + (1+time|IDPERS),
                   data=shp.lmem, REML=FALSE)

# Summary statistics of the model
summary(LMEM.model)


#####
# LCM

###############################
# Reshape data in a wide format
shp.lcm.data <- reshape(shp.lmem,idvar="IDPERS",timevar="time",
                        direction="wide",
                        v.names=c("SRH", "SATREL"))

# Load the package reshape that contains the function rename()
library(reshape)

# As the '.' is illegal for manifest variables in the function
# mxRun(), rename the variables SRH AND SATREL
shp.lcm <- rename(shp.lcm.data, c("SRH.0"="SRH0","SRH.1"="SRH1",
                                  "SRH.2"="SRH2","SRH.3"="SRH3",
                                  "SRH.4"="SRH4","SRH.5"="SRH5",
                                  "SRH.6"="SRH6","SRH.7"="SRH7",
                                  "SATREL.0"="SATREL0",
                                  "SATREL.1"="SATREL1",
                                  "SATREL.2"="SATREL2",
                                  "SATREL.3"="SATREL3",
                                  "SATREL.4"="SATREL4",
                                  "SATREL.5"="SATREL5",
                                  "SATREL.6"="SATREL6",
                                  "SATREL.7"="SATREL7"))


############
# Estimation

# Load the package OpenMx that contains the functions
# mxModel() and mxRun()
library(OpenMx)

# Specify the manifest variables' names
```

```
indic <- c("SRH0", "SRH1", "SRH2", "SRH3",
           "SRH4", "SRH5", "SRH6", "SRH7", "SEX",
           "SATREL0", "SATREL1", "SATREL2", "SATREL3",
           "SATREL4", "SATREL5", "SATREL6", "SATREL7")

# Create the model
LCM.model <- mxModel("LCM", type="RAM",
                     manifestVars=indic,
                     latentVars=c("B0","B1"),
                     mxPath(from="B0", to=c("SRH0","SRH1",
                                            "SRH2","SRH3",
                                            "SRH4","SRH5",
                                            "SRH6","SRH7"),
                            arrows=1, free=FALSE, values=1),
                     mxPath(from="B1", to=c("SRH0","SRH1",
                                            "SRH2","SRH3",
                                            "SRH4","SRH5",
                                            "SRH6","SRH7"),
                            arrows=1, free=FALSE,
                            values=c(0,1,2,3,4,5,6,7)),
                     mxPath(from=c("SRH0","SRH1",
                                   "SRH2","SRH3",
                                   "SRH4","SRH5",
                                   "SRH6","SRH7"),
                            arrows=2, free=TRUE, values=1,
                            labels="Ve"),
                     mxPath(from="one", to=c("B0","B1","SEX",
                                             "SATREL0",
                                             "SATREL1",
                                             "SATREL2",
                                             "SATREL3",
                                             "SATREL4",
                                             "SATREL5",
                                             "SATREL6",
                                             "SATREL7"),
                            arrows=1, free=TRUE,
                            labels=c("MB0","MB1","MSEX",
                                     "MSATREL0","MSATREL1",
                                     "MSATREL2","MSATREL3",
                                     "MSATREL4","MSATREL5",
                                     "MSATREL6","MSATREL7")),
                     mxPath(from=c("B0","B1","SEX",
                                   "SATREL0","SATREL1",
                                   "SATREL2","SATREL3",
                                   "SATREL4","SATREL5",
                                   "SATREL6","SATREL7"),
                            arrows=2, free=TRUE,
                            values=c(1,1,1,1,1,1,1,1,1,1,1),
                            labels=c("VB0","VB1","VSEX",
                                     "VSATREL0","VSATREL1",
                                     "VSATREL2","VSATREL3",
                                     "VSATREL4","VSATREL5",
                                     "VSATREL6","VSATREL7")),
                     mxPath(from="B0", to="B1", arrows=2,
                            free=TRUE, values=-0.0086,
                            labels="CB0B1"),
                     mxPath(from="SEX", to=c("B0","B1"),
                            arrows=1, free=TRUE,
```

```
                               values=c(-0.1349,0.0010),
                               labels=c("SEXB0","SEXB1")),
                 mxPath(from="SATREL0", to="SRH0",
                        arrows=1, free=TRUE,
                        values=0.0436,
                        labels="SATRELB"),
                 mxPath(from="SATREL1", to="SRH1",
                        arrows=1, free=TRUE,
                        values=0.0436,
                        labels="SATRELB"),
                 mxPath(from="SATREL2", to="SRH2",
                        arrows=1, free=TRUE,
                        values=0.0436,
                        labels="SATRELB"),
                 mxPath(from="SATREL3", to="SRH3",
                        arrows=1, free=TRUE,
                        values=0.0436,
                        labels="SATRELB"),
                 mxPath(from="SATREL4", to="SRH4",
                        arrows=1, free=TRUE,
                        values=0.0436,
                        labels="SATRELB"),
                 mxPath(from="SATREL5", to="SRH5",
                        arrows=1, free=TRUE,
                        values=0.0436,
                        labels="SATRELB"),
                 mxPath(from="SATREL6", to="SRH6",
                        arrows=1, free=TRUE,
                        values=0.0436,
                        labels="SATRELB"),
                 mxPath(from="SATREL7", to="SRH7",
                        arrows=1, free=TRUE,
                        values=0.0436,
                        labels="SATRELB"),
                 mxData(observed=shp.lcm, type="raw")
)

# Fit the model
LCM.fit <- mxRun(LCM.model)
# Warning message:
# In model 'LCM' NPSOL returned a non-zero status code 6.
# The model does not satisfy the first-order
# optimality conditions to the required accuracy, and no
# improved point for the merit function could
# be found during the final linesearch (Mx status RED)

# To take into account the warning message,
# fit again the model with starting values that are equal
# to the values estimated in LCM.fit
LCM.model.new <- LCM.fit
LCM.fit.new <- mxRun(LCM.model.new)

# Summary statistics of the model
summary(LCM.fit.new)
```

References

Baltes, P. B. (1987). Theoretical propositions of life-span developmental psychology: On the dynamics between growth and decline. *Developmental Psychology, 23*(5), 611–626.

Baltes, P. B., & Nesselroade, J. R. (1979). History and rationale of longitudinal research. In J. R. Nesselroade & P. B. Baltes (Eds.), *Longitudinal research in the study of behavior and development* (pp. 1–39). New York: Academic.

Bauer, D. J. (2003). Estimating multilevel linear models as structural equation models. *Journal of Educational and Behavioral Statistics, 28*, 135–167.

Bell, R. Q. (1953). Convergence: An accelerated longitudinal approach. *Child Development, 24*, 145–152.

Bell, R. Q. (1954). An experimental test of the accelerated longitudinal approach. *Child Development, 25*, 281–286.

Berkman, L. F., & Syme, S. L. (1979). Social networks, host resistance, and mortality: A nine-year follow-up study of Alameda county residents. *American Journal of Epidemiology, 109*, 186–204.

Bollen, K. A., & Curran, P. J. (2006). *Latent curve models: A structural equation approach.* Hoboken: Wiley.

Bryk, A. S., & Raudenbush, S. W. (1987). Application of hierarchical linear models to assessing change. *Psychological Bulletin, 101*, 147–158.

Carpenter, J., & Goldstein, H. (2004). Multiple imputation in MLwiN. *Multilevel Modelling Newsletter, 16*(2), 9–18.

Chou, C.-P., Bentler, P. M., & Pentz, M. A. (1998). Comparisons of two statistical approaches to study growth curves: The multilevel model and latent curve analysis. *Structural Equation Modeling, 5*, 247–266.

Collins, L. M. (2006). Analysis of longitudinal data: the integration of theoretical model, temporal design, and statistical model. *Annual review of psychology, 57*, 505–528.

Courvoisier, D. S., Eid, M., & Nussbeck, F. W. (2007). Mixture distribution latent state-trait analysis: Basic ideas and applications. *Psychological Methods, 12*, 80–104.

Cullati, S., Rousseaux, E., Gabadinho, A., Courvoisier, D. S., & Burton-Jeangros, C. (2014). Factors of change and cumulative factors in self-rated health trajectories: A systematic review. *Advances in Life Course Research, 19*, 14–27. http://doi.org/10.1016/j.alcr.2013.11.002.

Davidian, M., & Giltinan, D. M. (1995). *Nonlinear models for repeated measurement data.* London: Chapman & Hall.

Duncan, T. E., Duncan, S. C., & Strycker, L. A. (2006). *An introduction to latent variable growth curve modeling* (2nd ed.). New York: Routledge Academic.

Goldstein, H. (1989). Models for multilevel response variables with an application to growth curves. In R. D. Bock (Ed.), *Multilevel analysis of educational data* (pp. 107–125). San Diego: Academic.

Goldstein, H. (2011). *Multilevel statistical models* (Vol. 4). West Sussex: John Wiley and Sons.

Ghisletta, P., & Lindenberger, U. (2004). Static and dynamic longitudinal structural analyses of cognitive changes in old age. *Gerontology, 50*, 12–16.

Graham, J. W. (2003). Adding missing-data-relevant variables to FIML-based structural equation models. *Structural Equation Modeling, 10*, 80–100.

Graham, J. W. (2009). Missing data analysis: Making it work in the real world. *Annual Review of Psychology, 60*, 549–576.

Halford, C., Wallman, T., Welin, L., Rosengren, A., Bardel, A., Johansson, S., & Svärdsudd, K. (2012). Effects of self-rated health on sick leave, disability pension, hospital admissions and mortality. A population-based longitudinal study of nearly 15,000 observations among Swedish women and men. *BMC Public Health, 12,* 1103.

Laird, N. M., & Ware, J. H. (1982). Random-effects models for longitudinal data. *Biometrics, 38,* 963–974.

MacCallum, R. C., Kim, C., Malarkey, W. B., & Kiecolt-Glaser, J. K. (1997). Studying multivariate change using multilevel models and latent curve models. *Multivariate Behavioral Research, 32,* 215–253.

McArdle, J. J. (1986). Latent growth within behavior genetic models. *Behavior Genetics, 16,* 163–200.

McArdle, J. J. (1988). Dynamic but structural equation modeling of repeated measures data. In J. R. Nesselroade & R. B. Cattell (Eds.), *Handbook of multivariate experimental psychology* (pp. 561–614). New York: Plenum Press.

McArdle, J. J. (1994). Structural factor analysis experiments with incomplete data. *Multivariate Behavioral Research, 29,* 409–454.

McArdle, J. J. (2001). Growth curve analysis. In N. J. Smelser & P. B. Baltes (Eds.), *The international encyclopedia of the behavioral and social sciences* (pp. 6439–6445). New York: Pergamon Press.

McArdle, J. J., & Hamagami, F. (1996). Multilevel models from a multiple group structural equation perspective. In G. A. Marcoulides & R. E. Schumaker (Eds.), *Advanced structural equation modeling. Issues and techniques* (pp. 89–124). Mahwah: Lawrence Erlbaum Associates.

McArdle, J. J., & Hamagami, F. (2001). Latent difference score structural models for linear dynamic analyses with incomplete longitudinal data. In L. M. Collins & M. Sayer (Eds.), *New methods for the analysis of change* (pp. 139–175). Washington: American Psychological Association.

McArdle, J. J., & Nesselroade, J. R. (2014). *Longitudinal data analysis using structural equation models.* Washington: American Psychological Association.

McCulloch, C. E., & Searle, S. R. (2001). *Generalized, linear, and mixed models.* New York: Wiley.

Mehta, P. D., & West, S. G. (2000). Putting the individual back into individual growth curves. *Psychological Methods, 5,* 23–43.

Meredith, W., & Tisak, J. (1984). "Tuckerizing" curves. In *Annual meetings of psychometric society.* Santa Barbara.

Meredith, W., & Tisak, J. (1990). Latent curve analysis. *Psychometrika, 55,* 107–122.

Muthén, L. K., & Muthén, B. O. (1998–2012). *Mplus users's guide* (7th ed.). Los Angeles: Muthén and Muthén.

Muthén, B. O., Brown, C. H., Masyn, K., Jo, B., Khoo, S.-T., Yang, C.-C., & Liao, J. (2002). General growth mixture modeling for randomized preventive interventions. *Biostatistics, 3,* 459–475.

Nagin, D. S. (1999). Analyzing developmental trajectories: A semiparametric, group-based approach. *Psychological Methods, 4,* 139–157.

Pinheiro, J. C., & Bates, D. M. (2000). *Mixed-effect models in S and S-PLUS.* New York: Springer.

R Core Team. (2013). *R: A language and environment for statistical computing.* Vienna: R Foundation for Statistical Computing. Retrieved from http://www.R-project.org/.

Raudenbush, S. W., & Bryk, A. S. (2002). *Hierarchical linear models. Applications and data analysis methods.* Thousand Oaks: Sage.

Rubin, D. B. (1976). Inference and missing data. *Biometrika, 63,* 581–592.

Schafer, J. L., & Graham, J. W. (2002). Missing data: Our view of the state of the art. *Psychological Methods, 7,* 147–177.

Schaie, K. W. (1977). Quasi-experimental research designs in the psychology of aging. In J. E. Birren & K. W. Schaie (Eds.), *Handbook of the psychology of aging* (pp. 39–57). New York: Van Nostrand Reinhold Company.

Singer, J. D., & Willett, J. B. (2003). *Applied longitudinal data analysis.* Oxford: Oxford University Press.

Skrondal, A., & Rabe-Hesketh, S. (2004). *Generalized latent variable modeling: Multilevel, longitudinal, and structural equation models*. Boca Raton: Chapman & Hall/CRC.

Snijders, T. A. B., & Bosker, R. J. (1994). Modeled variance in two-level models. *Sociological Methods and Research, 22*, 342–363.

Snijders, T. A. B., & Bosker, R. J. (2012). *Multilevel analysis: An introduction to basic and advanced multilevel modeling* (2nd ed.). London: Sage.

Spearman, C. (1904). General intelligence: Objectively determined and measured. *American Journal of Psychology, 15*, 201–293.

Wainer, H. (2000). The centercept: An estimable and meaningful regression parameter. *Psychological Science, 11*, 434–436.

Chapter 9
The Analysis of Individual Health Trajectories Across the Life Course: Latent Class Growth Models Versus Mixed Models

Trynke Hoekstra and Jos W.R. Twisk

Introduction

Researchers in the field of life course research are often interested in analysing longitudinal data. One of the main advantages of longitudinal data is the possibility to study individual development over time (Singer and Willett 2003; Twisk 2013). Studying these individual trajectories for example helps to better understand how risk factors for diseases naturally develop throughout the life course and aids the understanding and unravelling of the aetiology of diseases, which is important for early detection and prevention. Several statistical techniques to study these individual trajectories are available, of which mixed models (MM) and latent (class) growth models (LCGM) are the most common. Both techniques aim to study

Parts of this chapter have been published as Hoekstra, T., Barbosa-Leiker, C., Koppes, L., & Twisk, J. (2011). Developmental trajectories of body mass index throughout the life course: An application of latent class growth (Mixture) modelling. *Longitudinal and Life Course Studies, 2,* 319–330.

T. Hoekstra (✉)
EMGO+ Institute for Health and Care Research, Amsterdam, Netherlands

Department of Epidemiology and Biostatistics, VU University Medical Center Amsterdam, Amsterdam, Netherlands

Department of Health Sciences, VU University, Amsterdam, Netherlands
e-mail: trynke.hoekstra@vu.nl

J.W.R. Twisk
EMGO+ Institute for Health and Care Research, Amsterdam, Netherlands

Department of Epidemiology and Biostatistics, VU University Medical Center Amsterdam, Amsterdam, Netherlands
e-mail: jwr.twisk@vumc.nl

C. Burton-Jeangros et al. (eds.), *A Life Course Perspective on Health Trajectories and Transitions*, Life Course Research and Social Policies 4,
DOI 10.1007/978-3-319-20484-0_9

(heterogeneity in) individual health trajectories, but do so in different ways. In short, MM are regression-based techniques designed to study the individual development of a certain variable over time by adjusting for the correlations of the observations within one subject. This is done by estimating the differences between the subjects; a variance for the intercept and a variance for the slope(s). The intercept is indicative for the baseline values and the slope(s) for the rate of development over time. LCGM also aims to study the individual development of a certain variable over time, but uses the data to additionally generate groups of individuals with comparable trajectories over time.

The purpose of this chapter is to explain and compare MM and LCGM in more detail by combining a methodological focus with empirical findings using existing life course data of the Amsterdam Growth and Health Longitudinal Study cohort. We will address practical issues with which researchers within life course research are confronted when aiming to find answers to their research questions, paying particular attention to when, how and why to use MM and LCGM. Further, detailed readings are recommended for interested readers (Hancock and Samuelsen 2008; Nagin and Odgers 2010; Nagin 2005; Preacher et al. 2008; Singer and Willett 2003; Twisk 2013).

The Amsterdam Growth and Health Longitudinal Study

In 1974, the Amsterdam Growth and Health Longitudinal Study (AGHLS) was initially planned to monitor the growth, health and lifestyle of groups of adolescents entering secondary school, over a period of 4 years (Wijnstok et al. 2013). The reason for this follow-up was a series of intervention studies to measure the effectiveness of more intensive and extra physical education lessons in 12–13 year-old boys (Bakker et al. 2003; Kemper 1995). In general, no clear effects were found. There were indications that large inter-individual differences between the pupils in biological development and habitual physical activity could have masked any intervention effects. At that time, health authorities were complaining about the level of fitness of youngsters in their late teens. In growing towards independence, the life-style habits of teenagers change considerably (with regard to physical activity, food intake, tobacco smoking and alcohol consumption). Thereby, their health perspective might also have changed. This illustrated that the teenage period is an important period in the life course. Because individual changes in growth and development can be described most precisely by studying the same participants over a longer period of time, the Amsterdam Growth and Health Longitudinal Study (AGHLS) was set up; approximately 500 boys and girls (mean age of 13 years) from the first two grades of two secondary schools in the Netherlands were included in the study.

In the first 4 years, the AGHLS was primarily aimed at the investigation of the natural course of dietary intake, physical activity and physical fitness as risk factors for cardiovascular disease, such as cholesterol levels. Subsequently, the

AGHLS was expanded with further rounds of measurements after the adolescence period, during the young adulthood phase. At each of these follow-up rounds of measurement, cardiovascular disease risk indicators and lifestyle variables were measured in a similar way to allow longitudinal comparison. Also, new, age-relevant measures for health and lifestyle were added to the test battery at each follow-up round. For example, when subjects were in their 20s, measurements of bone mineral density were added (Welten et al. 1994). In their 30s, the test battery was extended with, for example, carotid ultrasound measurements to determine large arterial properties to examine not only the 'clinical' cardiovascular risk factors but also the early preclinical cardiovascular damage (Schouten et al. 2011; van de Laar et al. 2012). In their 40s, microvascular function was added to the test battery as an even earlier indicator for vascular damage (Wijnstok et al. 2010, 2012). Moreover, to study the onset, timing and progression of neuropsychiatric disease, such as Alzheimer's disease, a magnetoencephalogram, a novel brain scan to assess communication of different brain sections, was added to the test battery (Douw et al. 2014).

During the adolescence period, participants were measured annually during school hours, and thereafter, six more examinations took place, of which the most recent took place when the participants were 42 years old. Currently, around 350 participants are still enrolled in the study. In 2013, a cohort profile describing in detail the Amsterdam Growth and Health Longitudinal Study was published (Wijnstok et al. 2013).

Focus of the Cohort for This Chapter

The substantive focus of this paper will be illustrated by body mass index (BMI), a well-known construct across many fields of research. Because this chapter focuses mainly on methodological issues, although by using empirical data, substantive findings will not be discussed in great detail. Interested readers are referred to the literature specifically focused on BMI, outside the scope of this chapter (e.g. Hoekstra et al. 2011).

For the analyses in this chapter we selected subjects who had valid measurements of BMI available at baseline (i.e. at age 13) *and* who had at least two additional valid measurements over time. In total, 378 subjects (51 % females) who were measured 3–10 times were included for the analyses presented in this chapter. Baseline characteristics of the sample are presented in Table 9.1. The sample size varies across the first four measurements because part of the sample was measured once during that period (Wijnstok et al. 2013). We performed the MM in MLWiN 2.30 (Rasbash et al. 2005) and the LCGM in Mplus 7.11 (Muthén and Muthén 2012) and first analysed the development of BMI over time for the whole cohort, and second we analysed differences in the development of BMI over time between males and females.

Table 9.1 Descriptive information (mean, standard deviation) regarding the development of body mass index

Age	Sample size	BMI (kg/m^{-2}), SD Females	BMI (kg/m^{-2}), SD Males	BMI (kg/m^{-2}), SD Study sample
13	321	17.81, 2.14	16.93, 1.42	17.39, 1.88
14	279	18.66, 2.08	17.68, 1.49	18.23, 1.90
15	272	19.41, 2.14	18.38, 1.66	18.95, 2.01
16	275	20.01, 2.10	19.21, 1.70	19.66, 1.97
21	131	21.65, 2.48	21.20, 1.67	21.45, 2.17
27	133	22.03, 2.36	22.46, 2.17	22.22, 2.28
29	125	22.46, 2.58	22.94, 2.22	23.70, 2.41
32	314	22.85, 3.13	23.79, 2.41	23.28, 2.85
36	300	23.57, 3.47	24.60, 2.68	24.06, 3.16
42	336	24.09, 3.87	25.20, 2.92	24.62, 3.49

SD standard deviation

Analysis of Health Trajectories Over Time: Mixed Models

When analysing health trajectories over time, we should take into account the fact that repeated observations of each individual in the dataset are not independent (Singer and Willett 2003; Twisk 2013). Simple regression analyses or analysis of variance are unable to fully incorporate these correlated measures and therefore, more sophisticated statistical techniques are needed to analyse these data accordingly. Several techniques to do so are available, of which mixed models (MM) are the most well-known techniques.

Model Assumptions

Mixed models have relatively straightforward underlying assumptions. Because they are regression-based models MM rely on the same assumptions (Altman 1991). Specifically, the residuals of the outcome variable should be normally distributed and in addition, the residuals around the (random) intercept and slopes should approximate a normal distribution. This can be easily assessed in any statistical software package. MM are also well suited in the case of unequal repeated measurements and the model assumes data to be missing at random.

The idea behind MM (Twisk 2013) was initially developed in the social sciences, specifically for educational research. Investigating the performance of pupils within schools, researchers realised that the performances of pupils within the same class were not independent (in other words; these performances are correlated). This type of study design is characterised by a hierarchical structure; also referred to as a multilevel structure. Pupils are nested within classes and classes are nested within

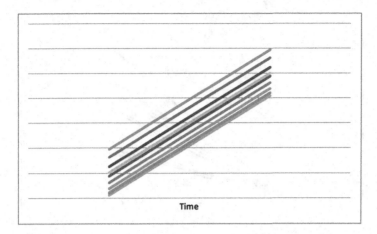

Fig. 9.1 Visualisation of different intercepts for each subject (random intercept)

schools. More or less the same structure is seen in longitudinal datasets where observations are nested within the subject: observations of one subject over time are correlated. MM adjusts for this correlation between repeated observations by modelling the variability among individuals through the inclusion of both fixed and random effects. To understand the general idea behind a mixed model, it is important to realise that with simple regression analyses adjusting for a certain variable (for example gender) means that different intercepts are calculated. In a longitudinal setting (thus adjusting for subject), this then means that for each subject, different intercepts are calculated. The simplest form of a MM takes into account this random intercept only. Figure 9.1 demonstrates that a model with a random intercept only allows the intercepts to vary across subjects. In addition to a random intercept, it is also possible that the *development over time* varies across individuals (indicated by a random slope). This is demonstrated in Fig. 9.2, where only linear slopes are assumed.

The Modelling of Time

Within life course epidemiology, MM are usually conducted to describe the development of a particular outcome variable over time (Beunen et al. 2002; Twisk 2013). In that case, the only independent variable of interest is a *time* variable, which can be included either as a continuous variable (indicating a linear development or other polynomial function of the outcome variable over time) or as a categorical variable. The modelling of time as a categorical variable allows for the incorporation of different developmental shapes during different stages in the life course, such as childhood, adolescence, adulthood and the elderly. This closely maps onto one of the focal points of life course research, which offers opportunities to understand the

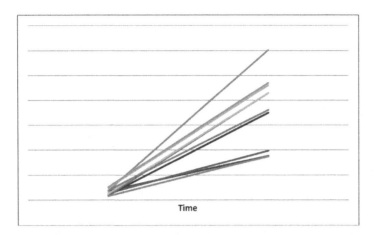

Fig. 9.2 Visualisation of differences in the development over time for each subject (random intercept and slope)

natural history of chronic disorders with a specific focus on health transitions and phases across the life course (Kuh and Ben-Shlomo 2004).

Comparing Models

Model fit of MM can be assessed by comparing the log likelihood values of neighbouring [nested] models. The likelihood ratio test (Bollen 1989) subsequently calculates the difference in -2 log-likelihood between two neighbouring models. This difference is assumed to follow a Chi-squared distribution with the number of degrees of freedom denoted as the difference in the number of parameters estimated with the two models.

Strategy and Results: Mixed Models

First, we will start by modelling a linear development of BMI over time. This model is relatively straightforward and includes the *time* variable as a continuous variable, which, in the case of the AGHLS would be 1, 2, 3, 4, 9, 15, 17, 20, 24, and 30. These values reflect the actual time between measurement rounds, taking into account the unequally spaced time points. Alternatively, ignoring the unequally spaced time points, this variable could also have values between 1 and 10 (one unit per measurement).

The simplest model includes a random intercept only. Table 9.2 demonstrates the results of this model and indicates that body mass index values are increasing

Table 9.2 Results of the mixed models

Model	Slope (SE)	−2 LL	Model	Slope (SE) Males	Slope (SE) Females	−2 LL
Linear			*Linear*			
Model 1	0.240 (0.003)	10,469	Model 1	0.285 (0.005)	0.200 (0.004)	10,288
Model 2	0.242 (0.006)	9,425	Model 2	0.286 (0.009)	0.202 (0.008)	9,367
Quadratic			*Quadratic*			
Model 1	0.436 (0.013); −0.007[a] (0.0004)[a]	10,244	Model 1	0.516 (0.018); −0.008[a] (0.001)[a]	0.368 (0.017); −0.006[a] (0.001)[a]	10,035
Model 2	0.443 (0.014); −0.007[a] (0.0004)[a]	8,753	Model 2	0.527 (0.019); −0.008[a] (0.001)[a]	0.368 (0.017); −0.006[a] (0.001)[a]	8,688
Life course			*Life course*			
Model 1		10,134	Model 1			9,916
Time2	0.936 (0.13)		*Time2*	0.788 (0.181)	6.277 (0.160)	
Time 3	1.677 (0.13)		*Time 3*	1.520 (0.183)	5.753 (0.165)	
Time 4	2.334 (0.13)		*Time 4*	2.344 (0.183)	5.088 (0.162)	
Time 9	4.046 (0.17)		*Time 9*	4.318 (0.237)	4.706 (0.224)	
Time 15	5.928 (0.17)		*Time 15*	5.633 (0.233)	4.286 (0.213)	
Time 17	5.400 (0.17)		*Time 17*	6.117 (0.231)	3.749 (0.212)	
Time 20	5.920 (0.12)		*Time 20*	6.871 (0.173)	2.255 (0.167)	
Time 24	6.654 (0.13)		*Time 24*	7.636 (0.173)	1.729 (0.167)	
Time 30	7.221 (0.12)		*Time 30*	8.253 (0.168)	0.982 (0.166)	
Model 2		8,026	Model 2			7,958
Time2	0.809 (0.04)		*Time2*	0.895 (0.059)	0.747 (0.065)	
Time 3	1.563 (0.06)		*Time 3*	1.622 (0.079)	1.487 (0.088)	
Time 4	2.212 (0.06)		*Time 4*	2.153 (0.087)	2.276 (0.097)	
Time 9	4.023 (0.13)		*Time 9*	3.711 (0.179)	4.350 (0.200)	
Time 15	4.893 (0.14)		*Time 15*	4.214 (0.184)	5.641 (0.199)	
Time 17	5.325 (0.16)		*Time 17*	4.552 (0.205)	6.176 (0.216)	
Time 20	5.960 (0.14)		*Time 20*	5.079 (0.185)	6.934 (0.195)	
Time 24	6.630 (0.15)		*Time 24*	5.711 (0.199)	7.642 (0.209)	
Time 30	7.204 (0.18)		*Time 30*	6.259 (0.234)	8.246 (0.246)	

−2 LL -2 log likelihood
Model 1: model with only a random intercept
Model 2: model with a random intercept and random slopes
[a]Parameters for the quadratic terms

over time. The regression coefficient for *time* for the linear model (model 1) is 0.240, so for each year, the BMI increases (linearly) with 0.240 kg/m^2. The corresponding standard error (0.003; indicative of the preciseness in the estimation of the regression coefficient – the smaller the more precise) can be used to assess the statistical significance of the regression coefficient by calculating the z-statistic (Altman 1991; Twisk 2013). The z-statistic is calculated by dividing the regression coefficient with the corresponding standard error. Values above 1.96 indicate statistical significance.

The next step is to extend the model with a random slope for *time,* indicating that the development of BMI over time is different for the subjects in the sample (model 2). These two models with a random intercept and a random intercept plus random slope can be compared by the likelihood ratio test to assess whether or not the inclusion of a random slope is necessary and improves the model fit. For each model, the -2 log likelihood is provided and although the value itself has no interpretation, the difference between two -2 log likelihoods can be used to compare neighbouring models. In our case, the distribution of the difference in the two -2 log likelihoods follows a Chi-square distribution with two degrees of freedom and this is highly statistically significant (i.e. $10,469 - 9,425 = 1,044$; this difference is much larger than the critical value). The result of the likelihood ratio test thus indicates that a model with both a random intercept and a random slope is significantly better than a model with a random intercept only.

These two relatively straightforward models assume that the development of body mass index is linear. It could also be possible that the development over time is better represented for example by a second-, third- polynomial function. Table 9.2 additionally shows the results of a model assuming a quadratic development (*time* as well as *time * time*) of body mass index over time. Whether or not this quadratic term is needed, can again be evaluated by the likelihood ratio test, or by evaluating the *P*-value of the regression coefficient of the quadratic term. The likelihood ratio test indicates a model assuming a quadratic development has better fit compared to a model assuming linear development over time and this finding is confirmed by a significant quadratic term ($-0.007/0.0004 = 17.5$, which corresponds with a $P < 0.05$). The interpretation of the regression coefficients is similar to those in a linear model, except that there are two coefficients to interpret; one for the linear slope and one for the quadratic slope.

Incorporation of Life Course Phases

The use of a 'straightforward' mathematical function in modelling the development of body mass index over time always assumes a particular development over time and does not necessarily take into account differential developmental shapes throughout the phases of the life course. A very elegant solution in this respect is to model *time* as a categorical variable instead of a continuous one. When *time* is modelled as a categorical variable, the development over time is modelled without assuming a certain shape in the development. Table 9.2 additionally shows the results of a MM analysing the development of body mass index with time as a categorical variable (represented with nine dummy variables – ten measurements). The regression coefficient for each of the nine dummy variables indicates the difference in BMI between that particular measurement and the first measurement, which is the 'reference' category. For example; the regression coefficient for *time 2* (0.936) is interpreted as the difference in BMI between the age of 13 and the age of 14. The positive coefficient indicates an increase in BMI. The corresponding model 2 demonstrates the same model, but additionally including a random slope.

Comparing Groups

Although the analysis of the development over time is of great interest, researchers are often interested in dividing the cohort under study into groups of subjects with comparable developmental trajectories; firstly as a tool to describe the population under study and, secondly as a first step to study either determinants or consequences of different trajectories. The possibility to divide the cohort under study within MM, however, is limited and only allows for the grouping of subjects into (predefined) categories such as gender. Categorisation into these predefined categories thus results in average health trajectories for each category, mostly assuming that each male or female has a similar health trajectory (shape). To do so, the interaction between the *time* variable and the *group* variable must be added to the model. Adding random slopes to predefined categories to the model makes it possible to model some heterogeneity within each category. However, this is not often done in practice, mainly because many software packages are not capable of performing such analyses. Table 9.2 shows the results of the MM analyses comparing the development over time between males and females. The interpretation of the numbers is exactly as has been given for the total population. All differences in development over time between males and females were statistically significant.

Although MM can allow for heterogeneity in health trajectory (shape) through the inclusion of random slopes, they only allow for the a-priori selection of subgroups of subjects. LCGM, on the other hand, relies on the data to generate latent subgroups of subjects with different health trajectories over time and consequently, potentially differential risks of disease. The application of such a 'group-based' approach, as opposed to the traditional 'classification-based' approach where subjects are classified into predefined groups is interesting for life course researchers too, because it allows the unravelling of distinct trajectories throughout the life course including their determinants and consequences and allows for the identification of high-risk subjects, who may need supplementary treatment or monitoring over the life course. Moreover, such an approach can also allow the subsequent identification of low-risk subjects who might need less attention.

There are several statistical techniques available to study heterogeneity in developmental trajectories using the data to form the groups; the most commonly used and the most flexible techniques available are probably those based on structural equation modelling (Bentler 1980; Bollen 1989; Kline 2005), i.e. *latent class (growth) models (LCGM)*. These models are actually extensions of MM and latent growth models (Preacher et al. 2008) and have recently been introduced in life course research (Dunn et al. 2006; Dunn 2010; Hoekstra et al. 2011).

Analysis of Health Trajectories Over Time: Latent Class Growth Models

Latent class growth models (LCGM) are extensions of MM and latent growth models (LGM). LGM are regression-based models that allow the analysis of observed and unobserved (or latent) variables. Latent variables are unobserved variables inferred from the data (Preacher et al. 2008).

Model Assumptions

LCGM also have relatively straightforward underlying assumptions, because they are also regression-based models. Specifically, the assumption of within-class conditional normality is important. This assumption assumes normally distributed measures within classes (Bauer 2007).

The observed variables are the body mass index measurements over time and the latent variables represent aspects of the repeated measurements over time. The most important latent variables are the intercept parameter and the slope parameters, analogous to a MM. The intercept also represents the initial, or baseline, status of the body mass index variable and the slope represents the rate at which this body mass index changes over time. In addition to the intercept and slope parameters, a LGM also models the variation, or variance around both these parameters. Similar to the random intercept and random slope in a MM, these parameters tell us something about the inter-individual differences; the larger the variance parameters, the more subjects in the study sample differ according to their initial status and/or development over time. Where in MM and LGM one single, average, trajectory is assumed to be sufficient to describe the individual trajectories (i.e. all subjects are represented by one underlying population), in LCGM one single trajectory is considered insufficient. This means that subjects in the study might come from multiple underlying (latent) subpopulations, with corresponding heterogeneity in developmental trajectory shape. The application of LCGM allows the (statistical) identification of the number, and characteristics (again, intercept, slope, and the variances around them) of these underlying subpopulations, hereby grouping the sample under study not based on predefined groups, but on groups (or classes) within the data. Thus, the subgroups to be revealed are latent. LCGM are also referred to as group-based models (Nagin and Tremblay 2001; Nagin 1999, 2005) and were first developed as the counterpart of the MM; both techniques aim to model individual-level heterogeneity in developmental trajectories but do so in different ways. In MM, we aim to describe the development of body mass index over time, incorporating heterogeneity within the sample. The main objective of LCGM is to statistically classify the subjects into distinct subgroups, each with their own growth parameters. In group-based LCGM, both the within-class intercepts and slope variances are set to zero (i.e. these parameters are not estimated), implying that subjects classified into the same class are very similar to each other regarding their individual trajectories. LCGM that do estimate within-class intercept and/or slope variance are latent class growth mixture models (Muthén and Muthén 2000) and imply larger within-class heterogeneity.

Choosing the Optimal Number of Classes; Comparing Models

Model fit of LCGM cannot be compared with the likelihood ratio test used in the MM example because from simulation studies it has become clear that the difference in -2 log likelihood does not follow a Chi-squared distribution and is therefore inappropriate (Nylund et al. 2007). Thus, other fit indices need to be used if we want to compare neighbouring models. The most often used fit indices are the bootstrapped likelihood ratio test (BLRT) and the Bayesian information criterion (BIC). The BLRT is also a likelihood-based test (McLachlan and Peel 2000), and overcomes the problems with the traditional likelihood ratio test. The BLRT uses bootstrap samples to empirically estimate the distribution of the difference in log-likelihood, hereby estimating the specific difference distribution. The test includes a Monte Carlo method involving the simulation of data and provides a P-value. A non-significant P-value would favour a model with one class less whereas a significant P-value would favour the other model.

The BIC (Schwarz 1978) is also used in MM and considers both the likelihood of the test and the number of parameters in the model, hereby penalising more complex models. A lower BIC value indicates a better fitting model, where a minimum on 10 points is often considered (Raftery 1995).

Choosing the Optimal Number of Classes Is Not Straightforward in LCGM

When conducting LCGM, model fit indices often do not consistently point to one best fitting model and the two model fit indices described in the previous section should both be considered. Although the BLRT has been demonstrated to be superior in choosing the optimal number of classes in simulated data (Nylund et al. 2007), in 'real' datasets this is often not the case and both indices should be considered. Moreover, because of the common inconsistencies, additionally, model parsimony (favouring the 'simplest' model), successful convergence, a minimum of 1 % of the study sample in each class, theoretical background and substantial interpretation of the classes (uninterpretable and theoretically impossible models are rejected) is taken into account too (Jung and Wickrama 2008; Nylund et al. 2007).

Finally, LCGM models are computationally-heavy models, often with convergence issues or hitting local maxima because of the complexity of the models. Random starts are recommended to avoid these issues as much as possible. In the current analyses, we applied 1,000 random starting values with 50 final optimisations. Only solutions with replicated log likelihoods were accepted. Because LCGM are complicated models, often problems arise when estimating more than three classes.

Strategy and Models: Latent Class Growth Models

Various LCGM models were run before choosing a final model. First, several linear LCGM with fixed intercept- and slope variance within-classes were investigated. Table 9.3 shows these results. The linear models are shown in the top four rows of the table, and point towards a three- or four class solutions. The interpretation of the slopes is the same as for the slopes presented in Table 9.2, only they are now class-specific; each class has its own estimated slope(s). For example, the slope of 0.269 indicates that for each year, the BMI increases (linearly) with 0.269 kg/m^2.

Next, quadratic slopes were added to the model allowing for curved developmental patterns as described in the section about MM. However, the quadratic models with three and four classes are increasingly complex and often result in untrustworthy output because of this complexity (e.g. negative variance estimates, difficulties with estimating other model estimates or classes with zero subjects (Jung and Wickrama 2008)). In our case, we had problems with the estimation of the quadratic slopes for some classes that appeared to include two individuals only. Therefore, for the quadratic models we had two models to compare to.

Incorporation of Life Course Phases

We subsequently investigated piecewise models which allow for different phases in development. Models with three pieces were investigated, showing possibilities of different growth rates (and directions) during each phase of the life course. Each phase thus has its own slope(s). Phase one was defined as the adolescence phase (age 13–16), phase two was defined as the young adulthood phase (age 21–27) and phase three was defined as the adulthood phase (age 32–42). The last rows of Table 9.3

Table 9.3 Results of the latent class growth models

Number of classes	Intercept	Slope(s)	BIC	BLRT	Probability	Subjects per class
1, linear slope	Class 1: 18.248	0.269	9899.165	Not calculated	1.00	336
2, linear slope	Class 1: 18.081	0.261	9884.609	i <0.001	0.930	324/12
	Class 2: 21.658	0.434				
3, linear slope	Class 1: 17.950	0.258	9887.077	P <0.001	0.863	310/10/16
	Class 2: 23.545	0.140				
	Class 3: 19.734	0.479				
4, linear slope	Class 1: 19.397	0.465	9894.435	P = 0.034	0.829	31/286/3/16
	Class 2: 17.757	0.259				
	Class 3: 25.537	0.267				
	Class 4: 21.344	0.119				
1, quadratic slope	Class 1: 17.809	0.436;−0.007[a]	8671.655	Not calculated	1.00	336
2, quadratic slope	Class 1: 20.661	0.530;−0.003[a]	8639.308	P <0.001	0.956	17/322
	Class 2: 17.663	0.431;−0.007[a]				
1, life course model[b]	Class 1: 17.442	0.743; 1.208; 0.538	8283.726	Not calculated	1.00	336
2, life course model[b]	Class 1: 17.292	0.752; 1.159; 0.497	8262.715	P <0.001	0.936	324/12
	Class 2: 20.892	0.515; 2.299; 1.528				
3, life course model[b]	**Class 1: 17.043**	**0.796; 1.130; 0.566**	**8265.720**	**P <0.001**	**0.867**	**297/24/15**
	Class 2: 20.160	**0.551; 1.514;−0.322**				
	Class 3: 20.924	**0.517; 2.313; 1.502**				
4, life course model[b]	Class 1: 19.498	0.681; 2.410; 1.294	8274.552	P = 0.05	0.910	16/2/294/24
	Class 2: 25.892	0.184; 0.824; 2.080				
	Class 3: 16.997	0.771; 1.116; 0.555				
	Class 4: 20.238	0.525; 1.431;−0.302				

[a]Parameters for the quadratic slopes

[b]Life course phase 1 (piece 1) is defined by ages 13–16, piece 2 is defined by the ages 21–29 and piece three is defined by the ages 32–42

show the results of these analyses. We see that the improvement of these models (specifically indicated by much lower BIC values) is clear.

The Final Model

Comparing the three sets of four models based on model fit alone was complicated, as often the different model fit indices are not in agreement with each other (Nylund et al. 2007). Based on the BIC, for example, the "best" model (i.e. the model with the lowest value) is the two class piecewise model, although the BIC of the three class piecewise model is almost the same (a difference of three points). Literature advices about "significant" improvement in the BIC-values; improvement of at least 10 points indicates a sufficient improvement of the model (Raftery 1995) indicating that based on the BIC, the two- and three class piecewise models have equivalent fit. Further, based on the BLRT, the "best" model is a four class model (indicated by a non-significant P-value). Both (BIC and BLRT) model fit indices therefore do not point consistently to one definite solution. Hence, we also took the substantive interpretation of the trajectories into account. We interpreted the meaning of the trajectories by assessing whether they make substantive sense. We assessed neighbouring models with similar statistical fit and rejected solutions that included classes that had no theoretically plausible meaning. Based on this, our final model was a three class piecewise model, showing a "normative" BMI trajectory (N = 297), a stabilising trajectory (N = 24) and a progressively overweight (N = 15) trajectory.

When the choice for the number of classes in the final model has been made, the necessity of random intercept- or slope variance within class can be assessed. This is done by additionally estimating one or more class-specific variance parameters for the intercepts and slopes. Subsequently, the model fit estimates as described earlier can again be interpreted. The results of these further analyses are not shown in the table, as none of the additional models showed a sufficient increase in model indices. Based on existing literature (Jung and Wickrama 2008) the ultimate final model was the most parsimonious model; a three class piecewise model without random intercept- and slope variance within classes (shown in bold in Table 9.3). Figure 9.3 shows the average trajectories of the final model.

Comparing Mixed Models and Latent Class Growth Models

Both MM and LCGM can be used to answer research questions that deal with the analysis of (heterogeneity in) individual health trajectories over time. Research questions dealing with the investigation of predictors for the development of a health- or disease marker over time, for example, can be analysed by means of a MM as well as a LCGM. However, although both MM and LCGM study individual

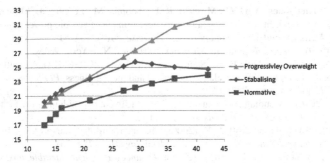

Fig. 9.3 Estimated trajectories of Body Mass Index (Y-axis) from the age of 13–42 years (X-axis)

developmental trajectories over time, LCGM classifies these individual trajectories into homogeneous subgroups based on the individual trajectories and MM relies on theory to create such homogenous groups, which are created a priori.

Conclusion

This chapter explained and compared mixed models and latent class growth models using existing life course data of the Amsterdam Growth and Health Study cohort. We combined a methodological focus with empirical findings and demonstrated the value of both techniques for life course researchers who aim to study (heterogeneity in) individual health trajectories over time. Both techniques can be used to study the individual development of a certain variable over time, but depending on the specific focus of the research question either LCGM or MM are preferred.

References

Altman, D. (1991). *Practical statistics for medical research.* Boca Raton: Chapman and Hall/CRC Press.
Bakker, I., Twisk, J. W., van Mechelen, W., Mensink, G. B., & Kemper, H. C. (2003). Computerization of a dietary history interview in a running cohort; evaluation within the Amsterdam Growth and Health Longitudinal Study. *European Journal of Clinical Nutrition, 57,* 394–404.
Bauer, D. J. (2007). Observations on the use of growth mixture models in psychological research. *Multivariate Behavioral Research, 42,* 757–768.
Bentler, P. (1980). Multivariate analysis with latent variables: Causal modeling. *Annual Review of Psychology, 31,* 419–456.

Beunen, G., Baxter-Jones, A. D. G., Mirwald, R. L., Thomis, M., Lefevre, J., Malina, R. M., & Bailey, D. A. (2002). Intraindividual allometric development of aerobic power in 8- to 16-year-old boys. *Medicine and Science in Sports and Exercise, 34*(3), 503–510.

Bollen, K. (1989). *Structural equations with latent variables.* New York: Wiley.

Douw, L., Nieboer, D., van Dijk, B. W., Stam, C. J., & Twisk, J. W. R. (2014). A healthy brain in a healthy body: Brain network correlates of physical and mental fitness. *PLoS One, 9*(2), e88202. doi:10.1371/journal.pone.0088202.

Dunn, K. M. (2010). Extending conceptual frameworks: Life course epidemiology for the study of back pain. *BMC Musculoskeletal Disorders, 2,* 11–23.

Dunn, K. M., Jordan, K., & Croft, P. R. (2006). Characterizing the course of low back pain: A latent class analysis. *American Journal of Epidemiology, 163,* 754–761.

Hancock, G., & Samuelsen, K. (Eds.). (2008). *Advances in latent variable mixture models.* Charlotte: Information Age Publishing.

Hoekstra, T., Barbosa-Leiker, C., Koppes, L., & Twisk, J. (2011). Developmental trajectories of body mass index throughout the life course: An application of latent class growth (mixture) modelling. *Longitudinal and Life Course Studies, 2,* 319–330.

Jung, T., & Wickrama, K. A. S. (2008). An introduction to latent class growth analysis and growth mixture modeling. *Social and Personality Psychology Compass, 2,* 302–317.

Kemper, H. (1995). *The Amsterdam growth study: A longitudinal analysis of health, fitness and lifestyle* (Vol. 6). Champaign: Human Kinetics.

Kline, R. (2005). *Principles and practice of structural equation modeling.* New York: The Guildford Press.

Kuh, D., & Ben-Shlomo, Y. (2004). *A life course approach to chronic disease epidemiology.* Oxford: Oxford University Press.

McLachlan, G., & Peel, D. (2000). *Finite mixture models.* New York: Wiley.

Muthén, B., & Muthén, L. (2000). Integrating person-centered and variable centered analyses: Growth mixture modeling with latent trajectory classes. *Alcoholism: Clinical and Experimental Research, 24,* 882–891.

Muthén, L., & Muthén, B. (2012). *Mplus user's guide* (7th ed.). Los Angeles: Muthén & Muthén.

Nagin, D. S. (1999). Analyzing developmental trajectories. A semi-parametric group based approach. *Psychological Methods, 6,* 18–34.

Nagin, D. S. (2005). *Group-based modeling of development.* Cambridge: Harvard University Press.

Nagin, D. S., & Odgers, C. (2010). Group-based trajectory modelling in clinical research. *Annual Review of Clinical Psychology, 6,* 109–138.

Nagin, D. S., & Tremblay, R. E. (2001). Developmental trajectory groups: Fact or a useful statistical fiction? *Criminology, 43,* 873–904.

Nylund, K., Asparouhov, T., & Muthén, B. (2007). Deciding on the number of classes in latent class analysis and growth mixture modelling: A Monte Carlo simulation study. *Structural Equation Modeling, 14,* 535–569.

Preacher, K., Wichman, A., MacCallum, R., & Briggs, N. (2008). *Latent growth curve modeling.* Thousand Oaks/New Delhi/London/Singapore: Sage Publications.

Raftery, A. (1995). Bayesian model selection in social research. *Sociological Methodology, 25,* 111–163.

Rasbash, J., Charlton, C., Browne, W., Healy, M., & Cameron, B. (2005). *MLWiN.* Bristol: Center for Multilevel Modelling.

Schouten, F., Twisk, J. W., de Boer, M. R., Serné, E. H., Stehouwer, C. D., Smulders, Y. M., & Ferreira, I. (2011). Increases in central fat and decreases in peripheral fat masses are associated with accelerated arterial stiffening in healthy adults. *American Journal of Clinical Nutrition, 94,* 40–48.

Schwarz, G. (1978). Estimating the dimension of a model. *Annals of Statistics, 6*(2), 461–464.

Singer, J., & Willett, J. (2003). *Applied longitudinal data analysis.* Oxford: Oxford University Press.

Twisk, J. (2013). *Applied longitudinal data analysis for epidemiology. A practical guide.* New York: Cambridge University Press.

Van de Laar, R., Stehouwer, C., van Bussel, B., te Velde, S., Prins, M., Twisk, J., & Ferreira, I. (2012). Lower lifetime dietary fiber intake is associated with carotid artery stiffness: The Amsterdam Growth and Health Longitudinal Study. *American Journal of Clinical Nutrition, 96*, 14–23.

Welten, D. C., Kemper, H. C., Post, G. B., Van Mechelen, W., Twisk, J., Lips, P., & Teule, G. J. (1994). Weight-bearing activity during youth is a more important factor for peak bone mass than calcium intake. *Journal of Bone and Mineral Research: The Official Journal of the American Society for Bone and Mineral Research, 9*(7), 1089–1096. doi:10.1002/jbmr.5650090717.

Wijnstok, N., Twisk, J., Young, I., Woodside, J., McFarlane, C., McEneny, J., & Boreham, C. (2010). Inflammation markers are associated with cardiovascular diseases risk in adolescents: The Young Hearts project 2000. *Journal of Adolescent Health, 47*, 346–351.

Wijnstok, N., Hoekstra, T., Twisk, J., Smulders, Y., & Serné, E. (2012). The relationship of body fatness and body fat distribution with microvascular recruitment: The Amsterdam Growth and Health Longitudinal Study. *Microcirculation, 19*, 273–279.

Wijnstok, N., Hoekstra, T., Twisk, J., van Mechelen, W., & Kemper, H. (2013). Cohort profile: The Amsterdam Growth and Health Longitudinal Study. *International Journal of Epidemiology, 42*, 422–429.

Chapter 10
Age, Period and Cohort Processes in Longitudinal and Life Course Analysis: A Multilevel Perspective

Andrew Bell and Kelvyn Jones

Introduction

Age, period and cohort (APC) effects represent three distinct ways in which health can change over time, and researchers across the social and medical sciences have long been interested in how to differentiate and understand these changes. First, individuals can *age*, meaning that they change as they progress through their life course. Second, change can occur over time due to differences between *cohort* groups, whereby as new cohorts replace old cohorts, the social composition (and thus the health) of society as a whole can change. Third, and finally, change can occur as a result of *period* effects, whereby passage through time results in a change in health, regardless of the age of the individual. Suzuki (2012, p. 452) demonstrates the difference between these with the following fictional dialogue:

A: I can't seem to shake off this tired feeling. Guess I'm just getting old. [Age effect]

B: Do you think it's stress? Business is down this year, and you've let your fatigue build up. [Period effect]

A: Maybe. What about you?

B: Actually, I'm exhausted too! My body feels really heavy.

A: You're kidding. You're still young. I could work all day long when I was your age.

B: Oh, really?

A: Yeah, young people these days are quick to whine. We were not like that. [Cohort effect]

A. Bell (✉)
Sheffield Methods Institute, University of Sheffield, Sheffield, UK
e-mail: andrew.j.d.bell@sheffield.ac.uk

K. Jones
School of Geographical Sciences and Centre for Multilevel Modelling, University of Bristol, Bristol, UK
e-mail: Kelvyn.Jones@bristol.ac.uk

© The Author(s) 2015
C. Burton-Jeangros et al. (eds.), *A Life Course Perspective on Health Trajectories and Transitions*, Life Course Research and Social Policies 4,
DOI 10.1007/978-3-319-20484-0_10

Understanding what combination of APC causes changes in health is of importance to many researchers, especially since different combinations of APC can have different public health policy implications. Unfortunately, meaningfully partitioning change into these three dimensions with statistical methods is far from straightforward, because age, period and cohort are exactly linearly dependent. This chapter considers the very serious implications of this 'identification problem' for longitudinal and life course research. Whilst the focus will be on health, the methodological and conceptual issues apply across the social sciences and beyond.

The chapter is structured as followed. We first outline the APC identification problem, and why simply controlling for age, period and cohort, as you might for imperfectly co-linear variables, does not work in the case of age, period and cohort. We show that the identification problem needs to be carefully considered whenever life course or longitudinal change is modelled, and that naïve models can radically reassign effects between age, period and cohort, producing misleading results. Next, we outline some proposed solutions to the identification problem, focusing on Yang and Land's Hierarchical Age-Period-Cohort (HAPC) model (Yang and Land 2006, 2013), and, using the example of the obesity epidemic, show how they often do not work. Finally, we outline what we consider to be best practice when considering APC effects, by extending the HAPC model, and demonstrate this with an example examining APC effects on mental health (measured by the General Health Questionnaire) using the British Household Panel Survey (BHPS). We argue that whilst there is no method that can mechanically separate APC effects in all scenarios, when good theory is used to make robust assumptions regarding APC effects, researchers can often make useful and non-arbitrary inference.

The Age-Period-Cohort Identification Problem

It is well known that in any dataset, the variables age, period and cohort will be perfectly correlated, such that[1]:

$$Age = Period - Cohort \tag{10.1}$$

As such, if we know the value of two of these variables, we will automatically know the value of the third. Consequently, when the true underlying process affecting a dependent variable includes linear effects of some or all of APC, there is a risk that we will pick the wrong combination, given that we could swap a term for the combination of the other two terms without changing the data. For example, take a contrived hypothetical process in which, say, an individual's level of health is affected by all of age, period and cohort, each with an effect size of 1:

$$Health = (1 * Age) + (1 * Period) + (1 * Cohort) \tag{10.2}$$

---

[1]This and the subsequent section are adapted from Bell and Jones (2014a), section "The Age-Period-Cohort Identification Problem".

Here, health improves (by 1 unit) as an individual gets older (by 1 year), improves for everyone as time passes, and is better amongst people who were born later. Substituting *Period* with *Age + Cohort*, we get

$$Health = (2 * Age) + (2 * Cohort) \tag{10.3}$$

And substituting *Age + Cohort* for *Period* gives us

$$Health = (2 * Period) \tag{10.4}$$

There will be no differences between the datasets generated by each of these three processes – they will be indistinguishable. There are important implications of this hypothetical illustration for researchers considering life course and longitudinal data. Say Eq. 10.3 was the true underlying process. Were we to estimate the effects found in Eq. 10.4, we would have erroneously found zero importance of life course processes, and found an effect of time that was simply not present. The modelling choices that individuals take will affect the results that they could find. A researcher may, for example, diligently control for a potential period effect (in the hope of estimating an unbiased age effect), and in so doing completely miss the very age effect (s)he was hoping to find. As such the APC identification problem should be a concern not just to researchers wanting to find all three APC effects, but to any longitudinal and life course researcher who wishes to model any of the APC effects robustly.

Unfortunately, there is no satisfactory solution to this exact collinearity. The problem is that the collinearity is present in the underlying process that creates the data and therefore in the population as a whole (not just in the sample). This means that neither a more sophisticated model, nor a larger dataset, will solve the problem. However as we see in the next section, a number of solutions to the identification problem have been proposed, many of which fail to understand the impossibility of what they try to do:

> The continued search for a statistical technique that can be mechanically applied always to correctly estimate the effects is one of the most bizarre instances in the history of science of repeated attempts to do the logically impossible (Glenn 2005, p. 6).

'Solutions' to the APC Identification Problem

The most common 'solution', and that suggested first by Mason et al. (1973), is to constrain certain parameters in a model to be equal.[2] Thus, each age, period and cohort group is entered into a regression model as a dummy variable, but two groups are combined as if they were a single group. This means that the dependency in Eq. 10.1 no longer applies (that is, it is no longer possible to

---

[2]This section is in part adapted from Bell and Jones (2013).

always be sure of the value of one of the APC variables if you know the value
of the other two). However, as Mason et al. recognised (but unfortunately many
who use the Mason et al. method do not), solving the dependency in the model
does not solve the dependency in the real world (Glenn 1976, 2005; Osmond
and Gardner 1989). Whilst the model will produce an answer, there is no way of
knowing whether that answer is correct unless we know that the constraint imposed
is exactly correct. Thus whilst saying that individuals born in 1960 are substantively
the same as those born in 1961 may seem innocuous, such an assumption could
have a profound effect on the estimated results, and produce very different results
from models using other apparently innocuous assumptions. Crucially, all of these
models will have identical model fit statistics, meaning there is no way of choosing
one constraint over another without strong prior knowledge. Other models use
similar constraints, for example using aggregated groups for one of APC similarly
constrains the parameters within those groups, for example see Page et al. (2013).
These models are subject to the same problem – the identification problem is merely
hidden beneath coarser data. Unless there is very good theory to believe that the
groupings imposed are exactly valid, the model will generally fail to produce correct
inference.

In recent years more solutions to the identification problem have been proposed.[3]
This section now focusses on one of these – Yang and Land's Hierarchical APC
(HAPC) model (Yang and Land 2006, 2013).

The HAPC model conceptualises period and cohorts as contexts in which
individuals (of a given age) reside. This structure makes repeated cross-sectional
data (that is survey data with multiple surveys over time) apparently suitable
to be modelled with a multilevel cross-classified structure (Browne et al. 2001),
whereby individuals are nested within cohort groups and periods of time, but periods
are not nested within cohort groups or vice-versa meaning a simple hierarchical
structure is not possible (see Fig. 10.1). Thus, the model is specified algebraically
as follows:

$$y_{i(j_1 j_2)} = \beta_{0 j_1 j_2} + \beta_1 Age_{i(j_1 j_2)} + \beta_2 Age^2_{i(j_1 j_2)} + e_{i(j_1 j_2)}$$

$$\beta_{0 j_1 j_2} = \beta_0 + u_{1 j_1} + u_{2 j_2}$$

$$e_{i(j_1 j_2)} \sim N\left(0, \sigma^2_e\right), \; u_{1 j_1} \sim N\left(0, \sigma^2_{u1}\right), \; u_{2 j_2} \sim N\left(0, \sigma^2_{u2}\right) \qquad (10.5)$$

The dependent variable, $y_{i(j_1 j_2)}$ is measured for individuals i in period j_1
and cohort j_2. The 'micro' model has linear and quadratic age terms, with
coefficients β_1 and β_2 respectively, a constant that varies across both periods
and cohorts, and a level-1 residual error term. The 'macro' model defines the

---

[3]For example see Yang's Intrinsic Estimator (Yang et al. 2004) which has been critiqued by Luo
(2013).

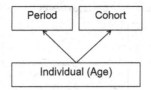

Fig. 10.1 Structural diagram of the HAPC model. Individuals, of different ages, are nested within periods, and within a cohort group. This is cross-classified because periods do not nest within cohort groups, nor vice-versa (Adapted from Bell and Jones (2014a) figure 1)

intercept in the micro model by a non-varying constant β_0, and a residual term for each period and cohort. The period, cohort and level-1 residuals are all assumed to follow Normal distributions, each with variances that are estimated.

This is an appealing conceptual design: "treating periods and cohort as contexts, and age as an individual characteristic, is intuitive to some degree because we move from one period to another as time passes, and we belong to cohort groups that have common characteristics, whereas aging is a process that occurs within an individual" (Bell and Jones 2014a, p. 340). However, Yang and Land go beyond this, arguing that this model does not incur the identification problem, because (a) the age effect is specified as a quadratic equation, and (b) because the multilevel model treats age differently from periods and cohorts:

> the underidentification problem of the classical APC accounting model has been resolved by the specification of the quadratic function for the age effects (Yang and Land 2006, p. 84)

> An HAPC framework does not incur the identification problem because the three effects are not assumed to be linear and additive at the same level of analysis (Yang and Land 2013, p. 191)

> This contextual approach ... helps to deal with (actually completely avoids) the identification problem (Yang and Land 2013, p. 71)

Unfortunately, Yang and Land are misguided in their belief in the HAPC model to do the logically impossible, as simulation studies have shown (Bell and Jones 2014a; Luo and Hodges 2013). Yang and Land's model can, and has, produced profoundly misleading results. For example, consider Reither, Hauser and Yang's APC study of obesity in the USA (Reither et al. 2009). They used the HAPC model to find that the recent obesity epidemic is primarily the result of period effects. However, simulations that we conducted (Bell and Jones 2014b) showed that these results could have been found when cohorts rather than periods were behind the increase in obesity. This is shown in Fig. 10.2 – data generated by us with a large cohort effect and no period trend (column 1) produced results suggesting erroneously that period effects were more important (column 2), in line with the results found by Reither et al. (column 3). The difference between these two possible sets of results are important from a policy perspective – a significant cohort trend would suggest that interventions should be targeted at young people in their formative years, whereas a period trend would suggest that interventions would be worthwhile for individuals

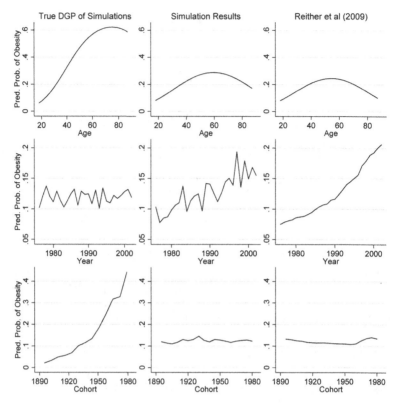

Fig. 10.2 (Column 1) The true data generating process (DGP) of simulated datasets; (column 2) the results from applying the HAPC model to those simulated datasets; and (column 3) the results found by Reither et al. (2009), for the age, period and cohort effects (rows 1, 2 and 3 respectively) (This figure is adapted from figure 1 in Bell and Jones (2014b))

at all stages of the life course. Additionally, the life course (age) effect found by Reither et al. differed significantly from that proffered by the simulations (row 1 of Fig. 10.2). Once again, failing to appropriately model period and cohort effects can have a big effect on the found life course effect, and vice versa.

How to Model APC Effects Robustly

Whilst the HAPC model does not work as its authors intended, it does offer a compelling conceptual framework which is useful looking forward to ways one might model age, period and cohort effects together in a single model without falling foul of the identification problem. We have argued from the beginning that discerning APC effects mechanically is impossible. However, if we are willing to make certain

assumptions about the nature of those APC effects, then inference is possible, and
the HAPC model provides us with a useful framework in which to do so.

These assumptions need to be strong: for example one of the APC trends is often
constrained to a certain value. The easiest way to do this is to constrain one of the
period and cohort linear trends to zero by including the other as a linear fixed effect.
For example, we may be willing to assume that there is no linear period trend, and
include a linear cohort fixed effect[4] in the model. Thus, Eq. 10.5 is extended to:

$$y_{i(j_1 j_2)} = \beta_{0j_1 j_2} + \beta_1 Age_{i(j_1 j_2)} + \beta_2 Age^2_{i(j_1 j_2)} + e_{i(j_1 j_2)}$$

$$\beta_{0j_1 j_2} = \beta_0 + \beta_3 Cohort_{j1} + u_{j_1} + u_{j_2}$$

$$e_{i(j_1 j_2)} \sim N\left(0, \sigma_e^2\right), \ u_{1j_1} \sim N\left(0, \sigma_{u1}^2\right), \ u_{2j_2} \sim N\left(0, \sigma_{u2}^2\right) \qquad (10.6)$$

We do not need to assume that there is no variation between periods in this model –
indeed the period residual term u_{2j_2} remains in the model meaning periods (and
cohorts) can still have contextual effects. However, we do assume that there is no
linear trend over time in the true period residuals, because these will be absorbed
by the age and cohort effects in this model.[5] If this assumption is justified, such a
model will produce correct inference both about the linear age and cohort trends,
and about the period and cohort random deviations from those trends (Bell and
Jones 2014a). We would argue that often constraining the period trend to zero
is a reasonable course of action. For us, the mechanism for long-run change is
more easily conceptualised through cohorts than periods – change occurring by
influencing people in their formative years rather than 'something in the air' that
influences all age groups equally and simultaneously. However, this is of course
dependent on the research question and subject area, and the researchers own
understanding of the process at hand.

Having made the above assumption, and thus (assuming the assumption is
valid) dealt with the identification problem, the model can now be extended in a
number of ways. First, using the multilevel framework, additional levels can be
added to fit the structure of the data being used. The HAPC model was originally
designed for repeated cross-sectional data (such as the ONS Longitudinal Study
(Office of National Statistics 2008)), where a cross-sectional sample of individuals
is measured on multiple occasions, but individuals are not followed through time
across these occasions. Where panel data (such as the BHPS) is used, that is
data that does follow individuals over time, an individual level should be included
to account for dependency within individuals between occasions. For other data

---

[4]Here we only include a linear cohort trend, but if we find it to be necessary we could additionally
include polynomials, as we do in the subsequent example.

[5]Where we are unwilling to constrain a trend to zero, but are willing to constrain it to an alternative
value, informative priors can be used in a Bayesian framework. See Bell and Jones (2015).

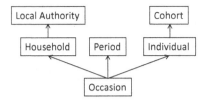

Fig. 10.3 An extension of the multilevel structure of the HAPC, for use with panel data and to incorporate spatial hierarchies. Thus measurement occasions are nested within individuals, which are themselves nested within cohort groups; measurement occasions are also nested into periods and households, the latter of which is additionally nested within local authority districts

designs, the HAPC model does not work so well: cross-sectional studies control for periods by design, but therefore cannot differentiate between age and cohort effects; whilst single cohort studies (such as the Millennium Cohort Study (Hansen 2014)) control for cohorts by design but cannot differentiate age and period effects.

In our example that follows, we use the British Household Panel Survey (BHPS) data (Taylor et al. 2010). Being a panel study, it follows individuals through time (in comparison to repeated cross-sectional data which selects a new sample with every wave), meaning that an individual level is necessary to account for dependency within individuals with occasions seen as nested within individuals. The BHPS also contains spatial identifiers (in this case, local authority and household variables), which could also help predict the dependent variable. Given this, it seems appropriate to extend the three-level structure outlined in Fig. 10.1 to a six-level structure shown in Fig. 10.3. Of course it may be found that one or more of these levels are not necessary and can thus be removed, but if all six levels were to prove significant, it would be important to include all of them to fully account for the dependency in the data and to assess the importance of individuals spatial, as well as temporal, contexts. It is certainly important to do this if one has potential predictors measured at a particular level.

Another extension would be to include an interaction between the age and cohort variable in the fixed part of the model. This is particularly useful for panel data, which effectively takes the form of an accelerated longitudinal design (for example see Freitas and Jones 2012). The age-by-cohort interaction allows for the possibility that the life course effect varies by generation – i.e. that there is not a single life course pattern that applies across all cohorts. In our view it is not appropriate to interpret this interaction as a period effect as others have done – for examples see Bell and Jones (2014c); the model still assumes that period effects are absent. The presence of an age-by-cohort interaction term is often thought of as a threat to inference about the life course, that is, a problem that needs to be corrected for (Miyazaki and Raudenbush 2000). However it seems to us that the interaction term can itself be of substantive interest, in understanding how life course trajectories have changed with changing cohort groups. Such an approach is increasingly common in the social medical sciences (Yang 2007; Shaw et al. 2014; Chen et al. 2010; Yang and Lee 2009), and in sociology more generally (McCulloch 2014). However, such designs are usually not combined with the cross-classified structure that characterises the HAPC model.

The model can be further elaborated by adding covariates at any level, or by allowing the effect of variables to vary at certain levels. For example, one could allow the life course (age) effects to vary between individuals, as is regularly done in simpler multilevel life course studies. One could also include control variables of various types, and interact these with the age and cohort variables to test whether the effects of these variables is constant over various dimensions of time.

The next section of this chapter puts this methodology into practice using the BHPS data to consider the life course and longitudinal effects on mental health.

Example: APC Effects on Mental Health with the BHPS

This example[6] uses data from the British Household Panel Survey (BHPS) to consider the age, period and cohort effects on mental health. The BHPS surveyed individuals from approximately 5,000 households (around 10,000 individuals) from across the United Kingdom (UK), every year between 1991 and 2008 (Taylor et al. 2010). These individuals are measured on a wide range of social, demographic, economic and medical characteristics. Here, our outcome of interest is mental health and to that end, we use the General Health Questionnaire (GHQ) (Goldberg 1972) to form our dependent variable. For the GHQ, respondents are asked 12 questions, and asked how far they agree with those questions on a four point scale. Each question is thus assigned a score from 0 to 3 on that scale, which are summed to create a single 36 point scale which can be treated as a continuous variable.[7] It is argued that the GHQ is a measure of psychiatric illness, both in terms of the severity of that illness, or as a probability of that individual being a psychiatric case (Goldberg and Williams 1988; Weich and Lewis 1998, p. 9), with high scores indicating a higher degree of psychiatric disorder. It should also be noted, however, that the GHQ is

---

[6]This analysis is a simplified version of that done by Bell (2014), which engages in more detail in the substantive debates about mental health, and uses further control variables and interaction terms.

[7]The GHQ is often assessed as a dichotomous outcome, where each question is scored as a 'case' or 'non-case' and respondents who are cases for 3 or more questions are considered cases overall. However, as Goldberg (1972, p. 1) states, "the distribution of psychiatric symptoms in the general population does not correspond to a sharp dichotomy between 'cases' and 'normals'. Psychiatric disturbance may be thought of as being evenly distributed throughout the population in varying degrees of severity."

"sensitive to recent change in psychological well-being" (Weich and Lewis 1998, p. 12) and "transient disorders, which may remit without treatment" (Goldberg and Williams 1988, p. 5), and as such also encompasses a subjective understanding of mental health that complicates an understanding of individuals being 'cases' or 'non-cases'.

In analysing this data, we first construct a 2-level multilevel model (with occasions nested within individuals). In this framework, age and cohort linear effects are included in the model as polynomials up to the cubic, with the highest powered terms removed when they were found to be non-significant. Here, we found evidence of a cubic age effect and a quadratic cohort effect. Next, we added a gender effect, and interactions between that and the linear age and cohort terms. We also added an interaction between the age and cohort linear terms (model 1 in Table 10.1).

Having established the significance of terms in the fixed part of the model, we then built up the random part of the model, to create the cross-classified structure portrayed in Fig. 10.3. A single level was added at a time, with the significance of that term assessed on the basis of a reduction in the Deviance Information Criterion (DIC) (Spiegelhalter et al. 2002). Our dataset contains 405 local authorities, 113,907 household years,[8] 18 years, nineteen 5-year cohort groups,[9] 25,889 people and 194,217 measured occasions, which form the structure of the random part of our models. In this case, it was found that all 6 levels were significant (the variances at these levels are different from zero) and were retained in the model (model 2 in Table 10.1). Finally we tested whether there were differential effects in the age effect between individuals, by allowing the linear age effect to vary at the person level; we also tested whether the random cohort variation was different for different genders, by allowing the gender effect to vary at the cohort level. We found the former to be significant and the latter insignificant (see model 3).[10]

---

[8] The BHPS does not provide data on households that is linked across time – that is, households are conceptualised here as transitory, changing each year.

[9] Cohorts were grouped into 5-year intervals in the random part of the model, to account for the autocorrelation between cohort years. However, single year groups were used to define the fixed part cohort trends.

[10] All models were run using Bayesian Monte Carlo Markov Chain (MCMC) estimation using MLwiN version 2.29 (Rasbash et al. 2014; Browne 2009), with a 500 iteration burn-in and 50,000 iteration chain length. For hierarchical models, starting values were obtained from Iterative Generalised Least Sqaures (IGLS) estimation (Goldstein 1989), whilst for the cross-classified models (which cannot be estimated in IGLS in MLwiN) the previous model's estimates were used as starting values, with small (relatively non informative) values used for any new parameters. To speed up convergence, hierarchical centering was used, which reduces the correlation between the parameter chains and so improves the mixing of the MCMC algorithms (Browne 2009, p. 401). All parameter chains were visually inspected for convergence, and the Effective Sample Size (ESS) was used to assess whether the model had been run for long enough. It was found that 50,000 iterations are sufficient to produce ESS scores of over 400 for all parameters. For practical advice on MCMC estimation see Jones and Subramanian (2013).

The results from three models – a two-level model, and two six-level models (one with random intercepts only and one with random slopes at the individual level on the age coefficient) – can be found in Table 10.1. As can be seen, model 1 (the two-level model) shows evidence of a significant age-cohort interaction with a negative coefficient estimate; this suggests that the life course effect is larger for earlier cohorts than for later cohorts. However this became insignificant when new levels were added to the model, and so in models 2 and 3 this term was removed.

Figure 10.4 shows the combined age and cohort effects on the GHQ score, based on the fixed part estimates of model 2. The cubic shape of the life course trend is clear, with an increase in GHQ score in young adulthood and in old age, but relatively stable GHQ score for the middle aged on average. The quadratic nature of

Table 10.1 Parameter estimates for the three models presented here. (1) A two-level model with age, cohort and gender specified in the fixed part of the model; (2) a six-level version of model 1; (3) as model 2, but with the age coefficient allowed to vary at the person level

	1. 2 levels		2. 6 levels		3. Age random slopes	
	Mean estimate	SE	Mean estimate	SE	Mean estimate	SE
Fixed part coefficient estimates						
Constant	10.934	0.046***	10.882	0.100***	10.922	0.111***
[a]Age (in 10-yr units)	−0.009	0.040	0.030	0.067	0.044	0.070
Age^2	−0.176	0.043***	−0.069	0.008***	−0.057	0.009***
Age^3	0.044	0.002***	0.044	0.003***	0.046	0.003***
[a]Birth year	0.008	0.004*	0.011	0.007 +	0.012	0.007*
Birth year^2	−0.001	0.000***	−0.000	0.000**	−0.000	0.000**
Female	1.322	0.052***	1.317	0.051***	1.279	0.055***
Female * age	0.051	0.042	0.053	0.043	0.043	0.047
Female * birth year	0.011	0.005**	0.012	0.005**	0.011	0.005*
Birth year * age	−0.021	0.008**				
Random part variance estimates[b]						
Local authority			0.160		0.142	
Household-year			2.458		2.425	
Period			0.015		0.015	
Cohort group (5 year interval)			0.057		0.059	
Person (intercept)	12.505		12.174		11.000	
Person (covariance)					0.077	
Person (age slope)					0.008	
Occasion	16.996		14.564		14.268	
DIC	1,120,612		1,113,079		1,110,445	

Note: + $p < 0.1$; * $p > 0.05$; ** $p < 0.01$; *** $p < 0.001$ (Bayesian p-values)

[a]Age and birth year variables in the fixed part of the model are all mean-centred. Age is in 10-year units, meaning coefficients are 10, 100 and 1,000 times the size for Age, Age^2 and Age^3 respectively

[b]No standard errors are reported for the random effects – these were judged significant on the basis of a decline in the DIC when added to the model

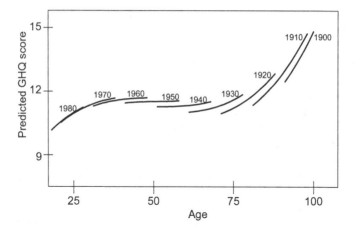

Fig. 10.4 Predicted GHQ score on the basis of cohort and age fixed effects (and so not including cohort random effects), from model 2. Each liner represents a different cohort group, with the label corresponding to that cohort's birth year

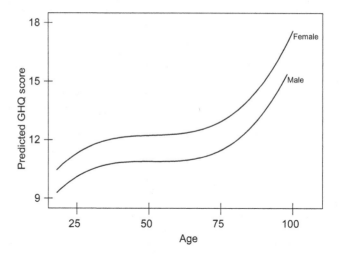

Fig. 10.5 Conditional age effect on GHQ score, for males and females, from model 2

the cohort effect can also be seen – more recent birth cohorts appear to report a worse level of mental health, but this effect is particularly pronounced (the lines are further apart amongst the earlier cohorts). However, in spite of its aesthetic advantages, this graph is actually quite difficult to read, especially in the presence of age-by-cohort interactions – it recombines the age and cohort effects that the model is aiming to pull apart and it is difficult to tell whether, for example, the 1980 cohort are of better health because they are younger or because they were born later. As such, Figs. 10.5 and 10.6 are somewhat more insightful – these graphs show the conditional effects of age and cohort respectively, that is the effect with the other variable kept constant.

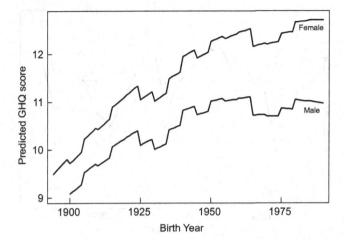

Fig. 10.6 Conditional Cohort effect on GHQ score, for males and females, from model 2. This is the combination of the linear and quadratic effects in the fixed part of the model, and the cohort random effects

Additionally, for these graphs we have separated the results by gender (utilising the gender-by-age and gender-by-cohort interactions in the model), and, in the case of Fig. 10.6, incorporated the random variation from the cohort level variance into the graph. As can be seen in Fig. 10.5, the male and female age trends are approximately parallel – that is, whilst women in general report a higher GHQ than men on average, this difference does not change through the life course (this can also be seen by the insignificant age-by-gender interaction coefficient estimate in model 2). In contrast, there are quite different cohort trajectories for men and women, with cohorts mattering more for women, and the gender gap in health being greater for more recent cohorts (Fig. 10.6). In other words, there is a general trend of recent cohorts being less psychiatrically healthy (or, at least, reporting lower levels of psychiatric health), and this is especially the case for women. Additionally, we can see that there were certain cohort groups in which individuals are in general more healthy than the general quadratic trend would suggest – the statistically significant ones (at the 95 % level) are the cohort groups 1930–1934, 1965–1969 and 1970–1974. This is an interesting finding – that, compared to the overall cohort trajectory, people born in these cohort groups are healthier – especially given that the groups fall onto two of the biggest economic recessions of the twentieth century in the UK. The suggestion of this is that, in the long run, being brought up during a recession is good for your mental health. It is worth bearing in mind, however, that these effects are relatively small compared to the overall cohort effect. We additionally tested to see if this between-cohort variation was different for males and females, but doing so did not improve the model; in other words there are no significant differences between men and women in the deviations from the fixed effect quadratic cohort trend.

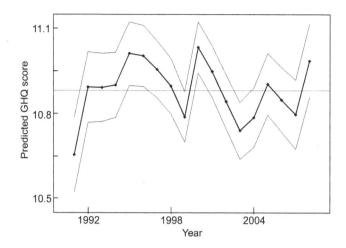

Fig. 10.7 Period effects on GHQ score (with 95 % confidence intervals), from model 2

Figure 10.7 shows the period effects – that is, the period residuals estimated in the random part of the model. These effects are in general small, although some are statistically significant at the 95 % level: people were in general healthier than average in 1991 and 2003, and less healthy in 2000.

Finally, model 3 in Table 10.1 shows that allowing the age effect to vary at the person level improves the model fit substantially (the DIC declined by over 2500). People differ in their life course trends of their GHQ measure, and this is expressed by the person-level coverage intervals[11] in Fig. 10.8. It can be seen that those with higher GHQ scores will experience a greater increase in GHQ scores over their lifetime than those with lower GHQ scores, and so the variance between individuals is greater amongst older people than younger people – this is a result of the positive covariance term (0.077) in model 3 of Table 10.1.

This model is for illustration only – one would normally add additional time varying and time invariant control variables (for example employment status, social position, income, wealth and ethnicity) in an attempt to account for the unexplained variation in the random part of the model. One could also further extend the model in any of the other ways mentioned above. It is also worth noting that, whilst this model presented here uses a continuous outcome, other outcomes could be used with different link functions (for example, if you wanted to analyse a binary health outcome, a logit or probit version of this model could be used).

---

[11]Coverage intervals are not to be confused with confidence intervals. The latter gives the uncertainty around a parameter, the former gives the expected variation for the data.

Fig. 10.8 Conditional
average life course effect,
with 95 % person-level
coverage intervals, based on
model 3. As can be seen, the
person level variance
increases with age – older
people are more variable in
their GHQ score

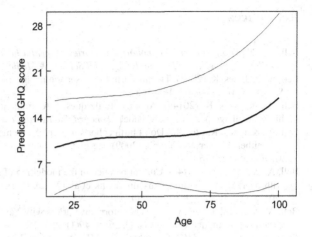

Conclusions

The aim of this chapter is to highlight the perils in modelling age, period and
cohort effects, and to provide some ways in which these perils can be overcome
in longitudinal and life course research, in health and beyond. We have shown
that researchers must put serious thought into which of age period and cohort they
believe are behind changes that occur in society, and these must be appropriately
specified in their model for accurate, policy-relevant inference to be made. We
have highlighted a number of attempts to disentangle APC effects, and shown the
shortcomings of these. Finally, we have presented a framework by which APC
effects can be robustly measured, so long as certain assumptions (in our case the
assumption of an absence of period trends) can be made. So long as this is the case,
both long run polynomial trends and discrete random fluctuations can be modelled
effectively, within a multilevel framework that can incorporate further variables and
levels. We do not claim that our most complex model is always necessary (indeed in
our example the simpler two-level model did a good job of accurately partitioning
APC effects); however undoubtedly the extendibility of the model we present here
is one of its strengths. Overall, we hope the chapter will encourage people to take
the APC identification problem seriously and, when investigating life course and
longitudinal effects, bear it in mind when constructing their statistical model.

References

Bell, A. (2014). *Life course and cohort trajectories of mental health in the UK, 1991–2008 – a multilevel age-period-cohort analysis. Social Science & Medicine, 120*, 21–30.

Bell, A., & Jones, K. (2013). The impossibility of separating age, period and cohort effects. *Social Science & Medicine, 93*, 163–165.

Bell, A., & Jones, K. (2014a). Another 'futile quest'? A simulation study of Yang and Land's hierarchical age-period-cohort model. *Demographic Research, 30*, 333–360.

Bell, A., & Jones, K. (2014b). Don't birth cohorts matter? A commentary and simulation exercise on Reither, Hauser and Yang's (2009) age-period-cohort study of obesity. *Social Science & Medicine, 101*, 176–180.

Bell, A., & Jones, K. (2014c). Current practice in the modelling of age, period and cohort effects with panel data: A commentary on Tawfik et al. (2012), Clarke et al (2009), and McCulloch (2012). *Quality and Quantity, 48*(4), 2089–2095.

Bell, A., & Jones, K. (2015). Bayesian informative priors with Yang and Land's hierarchical age-period-cohort model. *Quality and Quantity, 49*(1), 255–266.

Browne, W. J. (2009). *MCMC estimation in MLwiN, version 2.25.* Bristol: University of Bristol: Centre for Multilevel Modelling.

Browne, W., Goldstein, H., & Rasbash, J. (2001). Multiple membership multiple classification (MMMC) models. *Statistical Modelling, 1*, 103–124.

Chen, F. N., Yang, Y., & Liu, G. Y. (2010). Social change and socioeconomic disparities in health over the life course in China: A cohort analysis. *American Sociological Review, 75*(1), 126–150.

Freitas, D., & Jones, K. (2012). *Cohort change and individual development of aerobic performance during childhood: Results from the Madeira Growth Study.* Under review.

Glenn, N. D. (1976). Cohort analysts futile quest: Statistical attempts to separate age, period and cohort effects. *American Sociological Review, 41*(5), 900–904.

Glenn, N. D. (2005). *Cohort analysis* (2nd ed.). London: Sage.

Goldberg, D. (1972). *The detection of psychiatric illness by questionnaire.* London: Oxford University Press.

Goldberg, D., & Williams, P. (1988). *A user's guide to the general health questionnaire.* Windsor: NFER-NELSON.

Goldstein, H. (1989). Restricted unbiased iterative generalized least-squares estimation. *Biometrika, 76*(3), 622–623.

Hansen, K. (2014). *Millennium cohort study: A guide to the datasets.* London: Institute of Education.

Jones, K., & Subramanian, S. V. (2013). *Developing multilevel models for analysing contextuality, heterogeneity and change using MLwiN 2.2* (Vol. 1). Bristol: University of Bristol.

Luo, L. (2013). Assessing validity and application scope of the intrinsic estimator approach to the age-period-cohort problem. *Demography, 50*(6), 1945–1967.

Luo, L., & Hodges, J. (2013). *The cross-classified age-period-cohort model as a constrained estimator.* Under review.

Mason, K. O., Mason, W. M., Winsborough, H. H., & Poole, K. (1973). Some methodological issues in cohort analysis of archival data. *American Sociological Review, 38*(2), 242–258.

McCulloch, A. (2014). Cohort variations in the membership of voluntary organisations in Great Britain, 1991-2007. *Sociology, 48*(1), 167–185.

Miyazaki, Y., & Raudenbush, S. W. (2000). Tests for linkage of multiple cohorts in an accelerated longitudinal design. *Psychological Methods, 5*(1), 44–63.

Office of National Statistics. (2008). *ONS longitudinal study 1971.* UK Data Archive. Colchester: University of Essex.

Osmond, C., & Gardner, M. J. (1989). Age, period, and cohort models: Non-overlapping cohorts dont resolve the identification problem. *American Journal of Epidemiology, 129*(1), 31–35.

Page, A., Milner, A., Morrell, S., & Taylor, R. (2013). The role of under-employment and unemployment in recent birth cohort effects in Australian suicide. *Social Science & Medicine, 93*, 155–162.

Rasbash, J., Charlton, C., Browne, W. J., Healy, M., & Cameron, B. (2014). *MLwiN version 2.30.* Bristol: University of Bristol: Centre for Multilevel Modelling.

Reither, E. N., Hauser, R. M., & Yang, Y. (2009). Do birth cohorts matter? Age-period-cohort analyses of the obesity epidemic in the United States. *Social Science & Medicine, 69*(10), 1439–1448.

Shaw, R. J., Green, M. J., Popham, F., & Benzeval, M. (2014). Differences in adiposity trajectories by birth cohort and childhood social class: Evidence from cohorts born in the 1930s, 1950s and 1970s in the west of Scotland. *Journal of Epidemiology and Community Health, Online first.* doi:10.1136/jech-2013-203551.

Spiegelhalter, D. J., Best, N. G., Carlin, B. R., & van der Linde, A. (2002). Bayesian measures of model complexity and fit. *Journal of the Royal Statistical Society, Series B: Statistical Methodology, 64*, 583–616.

Suzuki, E. (2012). Time changes, so do people. *Social Science & Medicine, 75*, 452–456.

Taylor, M. F., Brice, J., Buck, N., & Prentice-Lane, E. (2010). *British household panel survey user manual volume A.* Colchester: University of Essex.

Weich, S., & Lewis, G. (1998). Material standard of living, social class, and the prevalence of the common mental disorders in Great Britain. *Journal of Epidemiology and Community Health, 52*(1), 8–14.

Yang, Y. (2007). Is old age depressing? Growth trajectories and cohort variations in late-life depression. *Journal of Health and Social Behavior, 48*(1), 16–32.

Yang, Y., & Land, K. C. (2006). A mixed models approach to the age-period-cohort analysis of repeated cross-section surveys, with an application to data on trends in verbal test scores. *Sociological Methodology, 36*, 75–97.

Yang, Y., & Land, K. C. (2013). *Age-period-cohort analysis: New models, methods, and empirical applications.* Boca Raton: CRC Press.

Yang, Y., & Lee, L. C. (2009). Sex and race disparities in health: Cohort variations in life course patterns. *Social Forces, 87*(4), 2093–2124.

Yang, Y., Fu, W. J. J., & Land, K. C. (2004). A methodological comparison of age-period-cohort models: The intrinsic estimator and conventional generalized linear models. *Sociological Methodology, 34*, 75–110.

Printed in the United States
By Bookmasters